# Contents

*The Basics!*

Do it Right!

# Part One
# Learning the Basics

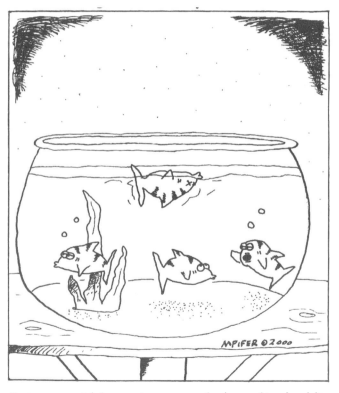

"Him? I wouldn't worry too much about him, buddy.
He does this every five minutes for attention."

# Introduction

Diagnosis and treatment of a fish disease is not, in itself, simple. The first logical step, though, is to equip yourself with the basic information of what species your fish is and what it needs to thrive. As a hobbyist, you should be aware of the common diseases that affect fish, as well as recognize how they show themselves and what you can use to treat these diseases.

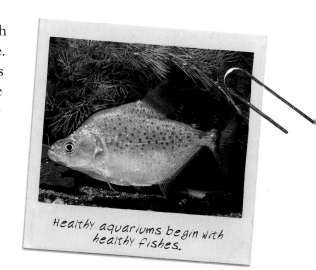

Healthy aquariums begin with healthy fishes.

If you know what species the fish is, you can then find out what environmental conditions it needs in order to thrive in captivity. Consequently, you will be able to compare these necessities with those things to which the sick fish is being exposed. This means that you can start to identify why an initially healthy fish has become ill and can begin to treat the disease. Possessing a familiarity with the common fish diseases that hobbyists encounter and recognizing what these diseases do to the fish will aid you in identifying the problem.

Once a likely problem is identified, you will be able to select an appropriate treatment. By correcting any underlying environmental or social problems (i.e. compatibility and interspecific aggression) and correcting them, you can attempt to prevent the problem from happening again in the future with the affected fish and any others you will keep further down the road. This book is designed to assist you in doing just that.

# The Five Freedoms

Fish do not become ill for no good reason, nor do they become ill to spite you or waste your money. Diseases are the result of an underlying problem. It may be an obvious problem, such as a super-sized male Malawi blue zebra (*Metriaclima zebra*) constantly beating up the other aquarium inhabitants, to something much more subtle, such as a fish tuberculosis granuloma slowly

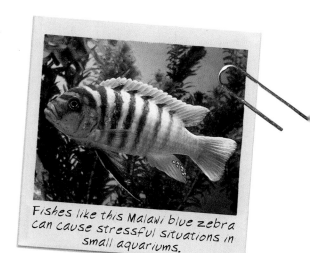

Fishes like this Malawi blue zebra can cause stressful situations in small aquariums.

eating away the inside of the liver (in which case the fish shows vague signs such as weight loss, abnormal behavior, and coloration). Regardless, there is always an underlying problem. Obviously there are some problems that we cannot realistically hope to predict, such as tumors in older fish, but there are plenty that we can, including the most common problem–STRESS!

## Stress

Stress means different things to different people, but in the context of this book I am going to define it as: *"An emotional and physical response to a given problematic situation."* I think that we can all identify with that, but if we look at this description further, we can start to see how stressful situations have an impact on fish.

### Emotional Response

This is the classic fight-or-flight syndrome. Fear, anger, and affection are examples of emotions that I would argue are displayed by some fish. I am not a fish and I am not one for being anthropomorphic, but to portray fish as simple stimulus-response creatures is, I feel, doing them a disservice. Of interest here is the fact that emotional responses trigger behavioral changes to deal with them. A fish swims away from a net, then, because it is frightened.

Rasboras will often form tight schools in response to a net being placed in their aquarium.

### Physical Response

This is what happens inside the fish to enable the emotional response. Hormones such as adrenaline and noradrenalin are released from adrenal tissue, as are natural steroids.

**Part 1**

These hormones speed up heart rate to improve the circulation to muscles, trigger blood sugar release from liver stores to fuel muscle metabolism, act as natural painkillers so that minor injuries will not impede any fighting or escape behaviors, and much, much more.

In nature, stress is often considered to be a good thing because it stimulates behaviors and physical changes that allow the fish to deal with any difficult situations that may arise. Prey species will attempt to swim away or hide from their potential predators. Fry-tending cichlids attack those animals that are considered as fry predators. Hungry fish will move on to new pastures. The problems arise when a stressful predicament becomes prolonged and the fish is unable to escape it, a situation all too common in the confines of an aquarium. Typical results of this are:

### Bullying

Dominant fish attempt to drive out competitors from where they feel is their territory. With several species, such as most large cichlids, their territory may be the whole aquarium. Because the other fish cannot physically get out of the aquarium (except by jumping, which does occasionally happen), then the other fish may become progressively more battered and oppressed. They may be unable to obtain sufficient amounts of food to grow properly or even survive, and consequently they gradually waste away, often succumbing to secondary infections in this weakened state. The dominant

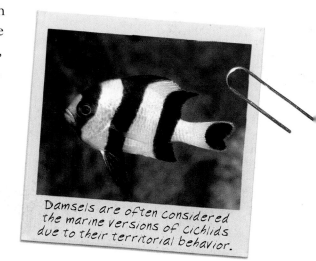

*Damsels are often considered the marine versions of cichlids due to their territorial behavior.*

fish, kept unnaturally on a high state of alertness and aggression by these constant intrusions into their territory, also become stressed and may show abnormal behaviors, such as attacking inanimate objects like heaters. Oscars (*Astronotus* spp.) are often guilty of this, as are red devils (*Amphilophus labiatum*) and midas cichlids (*A. citrinellum*) to name just a couple more.

### High levels of disease

Long-term high blood levels of natural steroids suppress the immune system, leaving the fish more susceptible to infection and disease. A working knowledge of the types of fish that you are keeping should allow you to tailor your aquaria and husbandry regimes more appropriately and avoid obvious stress factors. In addition there are five basic considerations that you can look at to provide for the welfare of your fish, thereby helping to avoid stress. These are the so-called Five Freedoms that were developed by John Webster (1995)[1]:

- Freedom from thirst, hunger, and malnutrition
- Freedom from discomfort
- Freedom from pain, injury, and disease
- Freedom to express most normal behavior
- Freedom from fear and distress

## Freedom From Thirst, Hunger, and Malnutrition

First of all, keeping your fish free from thirst is not usually a problem, but to provide a freedom from hunger and malnutrition means you need to address two main issues.

First, you need to supply enough food to them, and second, animals must feed in order to survive. Energy in the form of proteins, fats, and carbohydrates needs to be taken in to support all of the fish's metabolic processes, including growth, movement, internal organ function, and so on. Vitamins and trace elements are required for many of these functions, and most of these vitamins and trace elements will be derived from the food the fish eats. If you do not feed your fish enough food, it will be affected and you may see failure to grow, a lack of coloration, failure to breed,

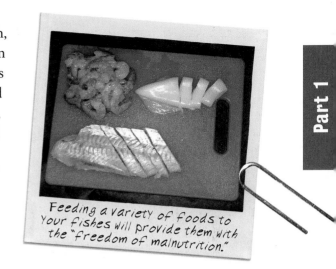

Feeding a variety of foods to your fishes will provide them with the "freedom of malnutrition."

and increased susceptibility to disease. Other causes of insufficient feeding include bullying, where subordinate individuals are unable to procure food because of the aggressive behavior of other fish in the tank.

Individual species variation should also be considered. Small carnivores and omnivores, such as tetras and many cyprinids (including goldfish), benefit from several small feedings a day, as this mimics their normal feeding behavior in the wild. Larger predators, such as the true piranhas (*Pygocentrus* spp.) and piscivorus cichlids like the wolf cichlid (*Parachromis dovii)*, will do quite well with alternate-day feeding because they are designed to take in large but sporadically available food items–remember, not every hunt is successful.

## Supplying the Correct Food

Offering frozen cyclops to adult Oscars (*Astronotus* spp.) is almost pointless, as is feeding frozen lance fish to a cardinal tetra (*Paracheirodon axelrodi*). These are extreme examples, but they work to make a point.

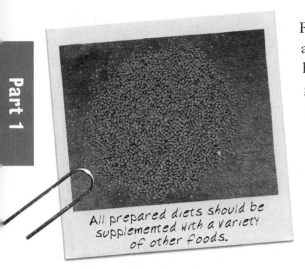

All prepared diets should be supplemented with a variety of other foods.

For the majority of ornamental fish available today, we are lucky in that we have commercially available shortcuts to good basic nutrition in the form of a wide array of flake, pellet, and tablet foods, some of which have been developed with individual species or groups in mind. For more finicky species, or to broaden the dietary range of easier kept fish, there is now a huge number of frozen foods one can choose from, including such things as bloodworm, *Daphnia*, and black mosquito larvae, as well as the various combinations marketed as discus foods, Malawi-mixes, and Tanganyikan-mixes. This doesn't even include the vast assortment of terrestrial foods, such as lettuce, cucumbers, and peas, to name just a few.

Some fish may require regular feedings of live foods, at least initially. Most often this is in the form of live invertebrates, such as brine shrimp, *Daphnia*, bloodworms, and even crickets. The latter will be happily shot down by the archerfish (*Toxotes jaculator*), grabbed from below the water surface by a leaping silver arowana *(Osteoglossum bicirrhosum)*, and skimmed from the surface by Boeseman's rainbowfish (*Melanotaenia boesemani*). Live food is often required for certain wild-caught fish, such as the Indian freshwater pipefish (*Ichthyocampus carce*), where movement of the prey appears to initiate a feeding response. However, over time it is usually possible to wean even these difficult species onto frozen foods. The following are two instances of feeding live food that I think need special attention:

• Live tubifex worms are enjoyed by many fish species. Unfortunately, a favorite habitat for these worms is in the mud of anoxic bodies of water. As a result, they may carry bacteria and other organisms harmful to fish, especially captive fishes under stress. Be sure of your source and keep them in a gentle flow of cool running water or else they will die and decompose rapidly.

• Feeding live fish such as feeder guppies or goldfish is in general not acceptable. First of all, there is rarely any need for it. Virtually all predatory fish can be weaned onto dead food. Secondly, there is a welfare issue, especially when the predator does not immediately kill the feeder fish. Such an example is the feeding of goldfish to small pirambebas (*Serrasalmus* spp.). Thirdly, it is an excellent way to pass on some really nasty diseases to your predatory fish, such as fish tuberculosis.

## Freedom From Discomfort

Water quality is the most obvious example under this heading. The minimum water quality testing should include ammonia, nitrite, nitrate, and pH. Other parameters, such as total hardness, carbonate hardness, and salinity (where applicable), may also be important depending upon which species you are keeping and whether you are keeping a freshwater or marine aquarium.

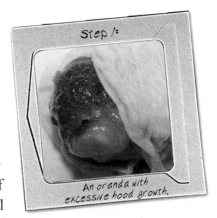

Step 1:

An oranda with excessive hood growth.

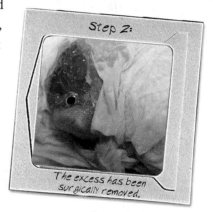

Step 2:

The excess has been surgically removed.

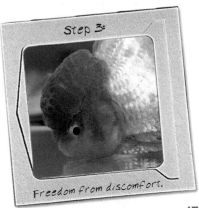

Step 3:

Freedom from discomfort.

Keeping to appropriate stocking levels also serves several functions here. Published stocking levels for ponds and aquaria are often calculated based upon surface area, filter area, or water volume. Regardless of whichever one is used, they allow for obvious essentials.

## Providing Sufficient Oxygen Levels

Dissolved oxygen levels in ponds in particular can vary widely over the year depending upon ambient temperature, circulation (pumps, fountains, and waterfalls), planting, and algal blooms. Calculations for pond stocking often seem extremely minimalist, such as 2.5cm of fish to 45 liters of water, but now you know why.

## Restricting Fish Numbers

This ensures that the filters can cope with the amount of total biomass, thereby preserving water quality. The bigger the filtration system is, the higher the stocking density that can be achieved. This is how wholesale and retail outlets are able to maintain such high fish numbers, often far in excess of that available to the home aquarist. These fish are often in aquaria that are linked to each other and so are actually in an enormous volume of water. These aquaria are, in turn, connected to a huge filtration unit.

# Freedom From Pain, Injury, and Disease

Pet fish should neither be exposed to potentially harmful objects such as sharp-edged dead corals placed in the aquarium for decoration (the fish are liable to cut themselves should they brush against it) nor placed with aggressive or predatory fishes.

Disease will strike in even the best-managed collection. Prompt action is essential both for the welfare of the individual fish but also to reduce the risk of any problem spreading to others in the pond or aquarium. Apathy and procrastination are common aids to a disease outbreak. One of the best defenses against infectious diseases in a collection is a period of quarantine.

Distasteful though it may seem, more intractable problems like tumors may require euthanasia of the affected fish. This also applies to terminally ill fish.

## Freedom to Express Most Normal Behavior

This is an important concept that is often overlooked. Fish are largely instinctive animals, with much of their behavior hard-wired into their nervous systems. Each species of fish has a behavioral repertoire with some room for learned behavior (such as associating the presence of people with food so that the fish dash to the surface in anticipation of a meal when their aquarium is approached).

By and large, however, their behavior is instinctive. This means that to a whole range of possible situations the fish may have a limited number of responses. As an example, if a fish becomes frightened, it's likely to either hide or to attempt to escape. What species of fish it is and where it evolved may have some bearing on which response it chooses.

A bottom-living, shell-dwelling cichlid such as *Lamprologus ocellatus* will attempt to hide, while the open-water *Pangasius* catfish (*Pangasius hypophthalmus*) will swim away; the surface-living marbled hatchet fish (*Carnegiella strigata*) will take flight above the water surface and land some

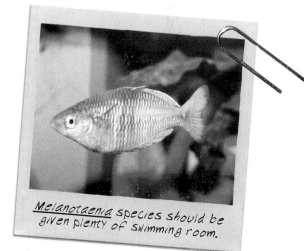

*Melanotaenia* species should be given plenty of swimming room.

Part 1

distance away. You can provide for the little shell-dwellers in a small aquarium, but the large, mid-water swimming *Pangasius* is liable to damage itself on the glass as it tries to dart away.

As for the hatchet fish, you should have a tight-fitting hood, although it may still damage itself as it ricochets off of the condensation tray. Thus, if you only had a small aquarium, then of the three species mentioned above, only the *Lamprologus ocellatus* would be really suitable, as in this situation it is the only one able to express its normal behavior.

Another example to be considered is that when two Texas cichlids (*Herichthys cyanoguttatum*) set up a spawning site, their innate programming will trigger them to defend an area several feet across and thus drive out other fish. This is an important survival strategy in their native habitat, as it provides a predator-free area of a sufficient size to provide food for their flock of rapidly growing fry. In a 4-foot-long aquarium, this same behavior is in force, but because any other fish present in the aquarium cannot physically leave the tank, this eviction behavior results in repeated beatings, stress, and often the eventual demise of the other aquarium inhabitants.

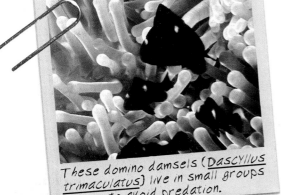

These domino damsels (*Dascyllus trimaculatus*) live in small groups to avoid predation.

## Safety in Numbers

Shoaling has many advantages for fish, but one of its most important functions is as an antipredation strategy. For example, if you are one of 100 fish, then there are 99 chances that when a predator attacks it will take one of your fellows and only one chance that you will become its dinner. Not only that, but if you can move faster and more athletically than your neighbor, then a predator is more likely to try the softer option of one of your less fit friends. Fish that naturally shoal, such as rainbowfish, tetras, and barbs, always do better in groups of three or more. It's a safety-in-numbers feeling that is good for their mental well-being.

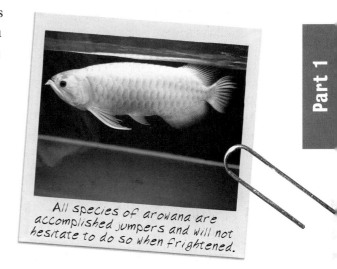

All species of arowana are accomplished jumpers and will not hesitate to do so when frightened.

Now consider a fairly active, shoaling fish that has evolved over tens of thousands of years to live in densely vegetated ponds and rivers and that spends most of its time grubbing around in the mud and silt of its native waters searching for insect larvae, crustaceans, and pieces of edible vegetation. That's right—consider the goldfish. Now put it in a bowl. This could be the ultimate example of the loss of freedom to express normal behavior. Okay, it may not *look* like a fish. It may have a double caudal fin, no dorsal fin, and a large sac of fluids sloshing around under each eye, but in its brain it's still a goldfish, and ichthyologists still refer to it as *Carassius auratus*. With care it will survive, surely, but that's really not the point.

## Freedom From Fear and Distress

Some of this has been touched on under the heading of normal behavior. Shoaling fish should have at least three, but preferably more, companions. Highly territorial fish either need aquaria large enough to provide individual territories or are best kept singly. Adequate hiding places of an appropriate nature should be provided. Rock-dwelling cichlids, such as many of the Lake Tanganyikan species, should have caves and crevices in which to hide. These would be of little use to freshwater stingrays of the genus *Potamotrygon*, which need fine sand in which to bury themselves should they feel threatened.

For pond fish there should be some protection from predators such as herons, cats, and the occasional overinquisitive child. Not only do these predators injure individual fish, but they also trigger stress and fear in the whole pond population. Many groups of fish, including the cyprinids (carp family) and characins (tetras and related species), release a chemical called "alarm substance" from their skin when they are damaged or injured. This chemical triggers predator-avoidance behavior in nearby fish–sometimes this can show itself as blind panic! Any skin trauma, whether it is from a heron attack or just poor netting technique, can cause its release.

These five freedoms are designed to give you an insight into the welfare of your fish. They all impinge directly on the health and well-being of the fish in your care. Remember that both physiologically and behaviorally, fish have very little room to change or adapt to new circumstances. If there is a problem you must address it, not ignore it and hope it will resolve itself. In my opinion, rehoming "problem" fish or euthanizing terminally ill fish is not cruel or an admission of failure but is an important aspect of managing the welfare of your fish.

[1] Webster, A.J.F. 1995. *Animal Welfare: A Cool Eye Towards Eden.* Oxford: Blackwell Science.

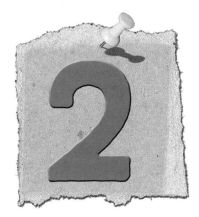

# Water Quality

The provision of good water quality is the foundation upon which all good fishkeeping is based. Good water quality is maintained by having an appropriate filtration system, performing regular water changes, paying attention to stocking levels, and feeding the proper amounts of suitable food. In addition, water quality testing should be performed on a regular basis. I would recommend a minimum of daily

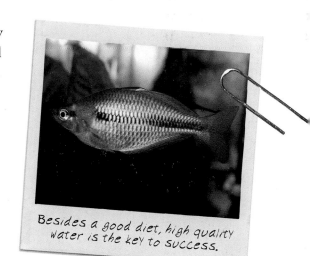

*Besides a good diet, high quality water is the key to success.*

checking of water temperature, weekly testing and recording of ammonia, nitrite, nitrate, and pH, with other values checked less frequently, such as carbonate hardness, general hardness, and oxygen levels.

## Temperature

Fish are ectotherms, which means that they rely upon the heat that they absorb from their environment to drive their metabolic processes. Fish are surrounded by water, and as they breathe, they are constantly drawing water over their gills. This means that any heat generated by their metabolism is lost very quickly to their environment; as a result, the body temperature of a fish tends to be nearly the same as that of the surrounding water. This does not necessarily mean that they are "cold-blooded." Gordon's platy (*Xiphophorus gordoni*), a native of hot springs, prefers temperatures above 80°F and can even manage 90°F. Even more interesting, bluegill sunfish (*Lepomis machrochirus*) are known for their ability to raise their body temperature above that of their surrounding water by basking in the shallows during cold weather, something that koi (carp) will do as well.

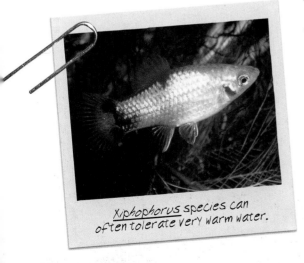

*Xiphophorus* species can often tolerate very warm water.

Water temperature is often overlooked with ornamental fish, and much of this has been due to the way that the hobby has historically classified fish as either "tropical" or "coldwater." Much of the original interest that sparked the phenomenal interest in keeping ornamental fish has been fuelled in northern Europe and the United States, both of which have marked seasonal temperature variations. If a fish needed no extra heat to keep it alive, it came to be described as "coldwater," and if it was from some exotic location and/or needed heat, then it was considered as "tropical." I believe that a more appropriate way of classifying ornamental fish by their temperature needs is to place them in three groups: true tropical fish, temperate-water fish, and true coldwater fish.

## True Tropical Fish

These are the majority of freshwater aquarium fish available in the hobby. Most of these are happy with a temperature range of 72° to 84°F although slightly higher temperatures are often favored for breeding. Some fishes are found in very warm water however, and the tropical aquarium temperatures are often towards the bottom of their preferred range. These natural waters are usually shallow and static, or with a very slow flow rate, and can easily reach

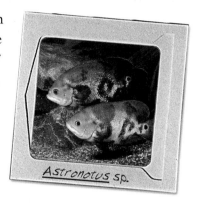

*Astronotus* sp.

temperatures above 86°F. Examples of these would be discus (*Symphysodon* spp.) and the chocolate gourami (*Sphaerichthyis osphronenoides*).

## Temperate-water Fish

These fish are from temperate latitudes or high altitudes and would include nearly all of the species from Europe, North America, and northern China. In their native countries, these fishes have to contend with wide seasonal temperature variations and must be able to survive the worst that nature can throw at them. However, these species do usually require higher (tropical) temperatures for breeding, and typically this would take place during their late

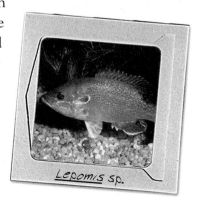

*Lepomis* sp.

spring or early summer months. Their ability to tolerate cold has led to many of these being erroneously classified as "coldwater," even though they prefer warmer temperatures. Typical temperate-water fish are goldfish, koi, and most other pond fish. Some aquarium fish also fall under this heading, including the paradise fish (*Macropodus opercularis*), the White Cloud Mountain minnow (*Tanichthys albonubes*), and the larger North American sunfishes (*Lepomis* spp.).

## True Coldwater Fish

There are relatively few species in this group in the hobby, but a common one is the sterlet (*Acipenser ruthenus*), which is regularly available as a pond fish. True coldwater fish are unhappy at temperatures greater than 58°F.

## Effects of Temperature on Fishes

If we think specifically about disease, then temperature becomes especially important because of its effects on how the fish functions and the changes in the surrounding water it can bring about.

### *The Fish Immune System*

Broadly speaking, a **fish immune system** has two parts–the cellular part that includes white blood cells and other hunter-killer cells that actively seek out and ingest pathogens or diseased cells, and a chemical part that consists of antibodies, along with other important compounds such as interferon and complement.

The various parts of the immune system function best at the fishes' preferred body temperature. It has been shown that in a well-researched fish, like the carp, its white blood cells have their highest activity and proliferation at around 83°F, falling off at temperatures above and below this point. Antibody production is optimal at 66° to 78°F, while carp that become infected at low temperatures (below 50°F) do not produce antibodies so long as they are kept at these temperatures. Worse still, some carp that are exposed to a minimal bacterial infection at low temperatures will become immunotolerant. This means that their immune systems will fail to recognize that particular disease-causing bacteria and thus do not mount any sort of immune response, even if the water subsequently warms up.

### *Metabolic Processes*

A great many metabolic processes in fish are temperature related. Just as with pH, the normal functioning of enzymes in the body depends upon the fish being within an optimal temperature range. Below this range, the enzymes will stop working, and above it they become damaged or denatured. Thus, if a fish is kept at the wrong temperature, its kidneys will not work properly, nor will its liver, and so on. As we have said before, fish have evolved in given habitats, and some even have a range of enzymes that work at different temperatures. This means that as the water gets warmer or colder, the enzymes that are used for a given function will change. In carp it has been shown that at low temperatures, certain genes become switched on, triggering the production of different enzymes that will work more effectively in colder conditions. Fishes that are able to survive over a wide temperature range, such as koi and goldfish, are known as eurythermal, while those that are dependants of narrow temperature ranges, such as discus (*Symphysodon* spp.), are called stenothermal.

## Effects on the Water

Increasing water temperature lowers the amount of dissolved oxygen present, which can cause serious problems, especially in heavily stocked ponds and aquaria.

Increasing water temperature will cause more of any dissolved ammonia to shift into the more toxic non-ionized form.

## The Nitrogen Cycle

This is basic knowledge of aquarium management and is a concept that helped to revolutionize fishkeeping. It is absent in many of the early (and not so early) books on ornamental fishkeeping.

A good place to start in the cycle is with ammonia. Ammonia is the end product of nitrogen metabolism in most fish and is excreted from the body through the kidneys and the gills. The main source of the nitrogen in this ammonia is dietary protein, and because most fish are carnivorous to a greater or lesser extent, most fish foods are by definition high in nitrogen compounds.

Ammonia excreted by the fish is changed into nitrite by a group of bacteria called *Nitrosomonas* that are present in mature biological filter beds and on other aquatic surfaces. The nitrite so produced undergoes a second conversion to nitrate by another group of bacteria–*Nitrobacter.*

Nitrate is considered to have two main fates. In some cases it is absorbed by aquatic and marginal plants and used by them as a food source, or it is converted to free nitrogen gas. This denitrification occurs in conditions of almost zero oxygen (hypoxic); in the majority of ponds and aquaria, this effect is very small.

"If a fish eats a plant or it eats another fish that has eaten plant material, then the nitrogen cycle has been completed."

The nitrogen cycle is an important concept because ammonia, nitrite, and to a lesser extent, nitrate, are all toxic to fish and so their removal from the water is essential for the long-term maintenance of fish in small volumes of water such as most ponds and aquariums. Biological filters, whether they are undergravel, trickle tower, internal, external, etc. are largely there to provide as large a surface area as possible for these bacteria to live on along with the high oxygen levels that they need.

Unfortunately, one must be aware that in the small volumes of aquaria and in many ponds, the nitrogen cycle does not happen. Nitrate is produced, but the next part, the uptake by plants and algae, does not happen to the extent that we are led to expect. This is obviously the case in aquaria where there are no plants, such as large Central American cichlid aquaria, for example. Most hobbyists want to keep fish, not plants, and so plants play second fiddle insofar as biomass is concerned (except in the most heavily planted Dutch-type aquaria). High levels of fish biomass mean high waste levels that can easily exceed the ability of the resident plants to cope. Even where plants are present, their usage of nitrate as fertilizer (as well as other substances, such as ammonia) depends upon the normal, healthy growth of those plants. This, in turn, depends upon other environmental factors, such as correct lighting (intensity, spectrum, and day length), pH, hardness, iron availability, and so on. In most home aquaria, plants do not thrive–they subsist. Also, we buy plants to adorn our tanks and ponds, not to act as a (healthy) dietary supplement. If the fish do eat them, we tend to either change the fish or swap to plastic plants.

It is only in well-planted ponds and aquaria with low stocking densities will anything close to a true nitrogen cycle have an opportunity to take place. For most of us, we control nitrate levels either by regular water changes or by using nitrate absorbers–various resins placed into the filtration compartments that lock up any nitrate present. These resins need to be changed on a regular basis.

## Ammonia

Ammonia is produced as the major waste product of most fish. Ammonia is very water-soluble and is actively excreted by the kidneys in urine and by the gills. In nature, the ammonia released into the surrounding water is diluted to infinitesimal levels by the surrounding larger volumes of water.

When the ammonia molecule dissolves in water, it picks up an extra hydrogen atom to form the ammonium. This gives it an extra positive charge, and the ammonia is considered ionized. It is now known as the ammonium ion.

$$NH_3 \quad + \quad H_2O \quad \Longleftrightarrow \quad NH_4^+ \quad + \quad OH^-$$
(Ammonia)    (Water)    (Ammonium ion)    (Hydroxyl ion)

This is not a one-way equation. It is an equilibrium that is constantly trying to balance itself. Therefore, if we load more ammonia, the equation shifts to the right, producing more ammonium. If we load more ammonium, the reverse happens. This gives us the idea of measuring the total ammonia levels, which in turn is what we get when we add the non-ionized ammonia levels to the ionized ammonium levels. Environmental factors can cause the equation to go either way. Common factors are temperature, pH, and salinity.

Ammonia in both of its forms is toxic. However, the extra charge on the ammonium ion stops it from crossing certain molecular barriers in the body (such as those between the blood and the brain), thus reducing its toxicity. This is not the case with non-ionized ammonia, as it is able to cross these barriers with ease, causing damage to internal organs (especially the central nervous system, where it can trigger obvious behavioral disorders). It can be an irritant as well, causing some thickening of gill tissue and irritation to the skin.

Dissolved ammonia levels are controlled in most systems by cultivating large colonies of the beneficial *Nitrosomonas* bacteria in the filtration system, which

**Part 1**

"feed" on ammonia, converting it to the less toxic nitrite. Safe levels of total ammonia are considered to be less than 0.02mg/l. A large variety of test kits are available for measuring ammonia levels. Some will even give a conversion table to work out the percentage of non-ionized versus ionized levels. Factors that lead to dangerous levels of ammonia are poor husbandry, rapid overstocking, and filter insufficiencies. Rift Lake aquaria, with their tropical temperatures and high pH, are particularly at risk.

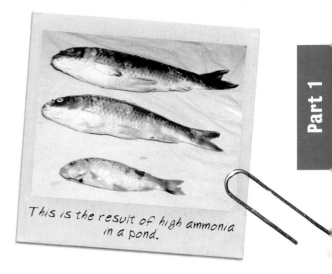

This is the result of high ammonia in a pond.

Chloramines are another potential source. This is a chemical combination of ammonia and chlorine that is added by some water companies as an antibacterial agent to tap water. It is more persistent than chlorine but will eventually break down into its component parts.

All species are susceptible, although some may be more tolerant than others. In one study, goldfish were unaffected by total ammonia levels of 0.025mg/l, but 10% died within 24 hours at 0.04mg/l. Affected fish stopped swimming, settled on the bottom, and eventually turned on to their sides, forming a "U" shape. Breathing movements slowed progressively until death occurred. Even at a late stage, some goldfish were able to recover if placed into ammonia-free water.

In ponds and aquaria with ammonia poisoning, all of the fish are likely to be affected. Common signs include loss of appetite and obvious behavioral abnormalities, such as thrashing around and heavy breathing indicating marked respiratory distress. The fish may produce excess mucus, and unexpected deaths may also occur. Many of these signs are similar to those seen with other water-quality problems or ectoparasitic diseases, so attempt to rule these out. Even moderately low levels of ammonia over a period of time can cause problems, such as reduced growth rate and increased disease susceptibility.

Deal with ammonia poisoning by transferring the fish to identical but ammonia-free water (e.g. to another aquarium) if this is at all possible. If this is not possible, then instigate partial water changes to dilute the ammonia concentration. In freshwater aquaria and ponds, the mineral zeolite will absorb large quantities of ammonia. Longer-term control may include the addition of commercially available *Nitrosomonas* bacterial cultures or an equivalent.

## Nitrite

*Nitrosomonas* bacteria produce nitrite from ammonia. It is absorbed from the surrounding water by these bacteria, where it is used in their internal biochemical reactions.

It is by this process that ammonia is converted to nitrite, which in turn is released into the water. Temperature and pH have no direct effect on the chemical process, other than any effects they may have on the *Nitrosomonas* bacteria directly. In a mature filter, *Nitrobacter* convert nitrite into nitrate by a similar process, preventing dangerous increases in nitrite level.

Problems arise when levels start to rise above 0.2mg/l. Nitrite is absorbed across the gills and is taken into the red blood cells. Here it combines with the oxygen-carrying pigment hemoglobin to form the stable compound methemoglobin. In this form hemoglobin cannot carry oxygen, and once significant numbers of red blood cells are affected, the fish is unable to supply its body with enough oxygen to survive. Normal hemoglobin is red, but methemoglobin is brown, so affected fish often show brownish-red coloration to the gills instead of a more normal reddish-pink. Natural recovery can only occur by replacement of these methemoglobin carrying red blood cells with new, unaffected ones.

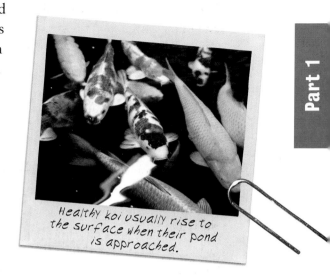

*Healthy koi usually rise to the surface when their pond is approached.*

Fish that are exposed to long-term low nitrite levels can become anemic and are predisposed to secondary infections. Seriously affected fish will show respiratory distress and gasp at the surface. Commonly, they congregate around filter outlets, where instinct tells them that oxygen levels are highest. Nitrite levels above 0.5mg/l can be fatal.

Nitrite poisoning can occur with any situation that promotes the production of large quantities of ammonia that can then be converted to nitrite, or any situation that stops the conversion of nitrite to nitrate. This would include overfeeding, overstocking, rotting plants, and other debris. Immature filters may lack enough *Nitrobacter* colonies to work properly, or exposure to low temperatures may shut down bacterial metabolism, preventing bacterial conversion of nitrite.

All species are susceptible, although some species are able to tolerate higher levels than others can. The typical sign is respiratory distress. The gills may appear brownish colored. Some fish—the classic being tiger barbs (*Puntius tetrazona*)—adopt a head-standing position in the water. Standard nitrite tests will pick up significant nitrite levels if they are present.

In severe cases, adding salt to the water to a concentration of 0.3%, the equivalent of 3.0kg per 1000 liters, can be beneficial. This is because the chloride ions from salt (sodium chloride) compete with nitrite ions at the gills where nitrite enters, reducing the number of nitrite ions absorbed. Otherwise, partial water changes are needed to dilute the nitrite levels down, combined with an overall assessment of stocking levels, feeding practices, and so on. Adding extra bacterial cultures in the form of commercially available freeze-dried or suspended cultures may be of some benefit. It has been suggested that dietary vitamin C may have a protective function, although its effect is less than that of salt.

*High nitrate concentrations arise through two main scenarios:*

**• Long-Term Environmental Buildup**

Assuming your biological filtration is working well, all nitrite that is passed through the *Nitrobacter*-laden media will be converted to nitrate. High stocking densities, high feeding rates, and decomposing fish and plants will all contribute. Failure to undertake regular water changes of sufficient volume will also ail a progressive overall increase.

**• High Ambient Tap Water Levels**

In some areas these can be very high, and if you are having chronic problems with nitrate levels then it is worth double-checking on your tap water.

Nitrate levels can be controlled and reduced by regular water changes with low nitrate water. Reverse osmosis (R.O.) water is an ideal means of providing zero nitrate water in those areas with high tap water nitrate levels. This is virtually pure water and so does need mixing with some normal tap water or buffering agents before use in order to increase the hardness to fish-friendly levels.

Although affected fish will be exhibiting apparent breathing problems, vigorous aeration may not help as much as you expect because the problem is with the fishes' ability to carry oxygen in their blood, not low oxygen levels in the water. However, increasing oxygen levels as much as possible will help the fish to make the best use of what oxygen they have access to. Nitrite testing kits are readily available, so the diagnosis of the problem is usually fairly straightforward.

Other water-quality problems can mimic this condition (especially those causing gill disorders such as ammonia poisoning). Also, gill diseases, such as severe gill fluke infestations, bacterial gill disease, and fungal infections, can result from poor water quality. Certain medications, such as malachite green, can mimic nitrite poisoning if present in excess, too.

## Nitrate

In many books, nitrate is described as non-toxic. This simply is not true. Its actions are often more subtle, and as a result, less well studied than ammonia and nitrite, but they do occur. Certainly high levels appear to act as stressors, and it is thought that at high concentrations nitrate may have an osmotic effect.

Suggested minimum lethal levels are 50.0 to 300.0mg/liter for sensitive fish. Even the bombproof goldfish has an experimental upper limit of 1,600.0mg/l.

## Vegetable Filters

Many pond owners allow the water discharge from their filters to pass through a section that is heavily planted, especially with "greedy" plants such as watercress. These plants are able to utilize nitrates as fertilizer. Heavy planting of aquaria may have a similar effect.

## Denitrators

These are biological filters that cultivate anaerobic bacteria to convert nitrate into free nitrogen, which then dissipates at the water surface. Denitrators are used primarily with marine invertebrate aquariums, as they are unlikely to be able to cope with the nitrate output of large numbers of fish.

Regular testing with commercially available test kits is the best way to monitor nitrate levels. Recommended levels obviously vary according to your aquarium inhabitants; aim for values less than 40.0mg/l. If your tap water levels are high, then aim not to exceed 40.0mg/l above the level normally found in your tap water, or use low nitrate water such as that produced by reverse osmosis.

"There are also some denitrating products available to add to your aquarium through pet shops and aquarium supply outlets. Use caution with these products, however, because they tend to evoke a sort of laziness among hobbyists. Remember, if you have poor water it's best to remove it and add water of good quality."

## pH

pH is a measurement of how *acidic* a given sample of water is. The opposite of acidic is *alkaline*. pH is measured on a scale of 0.0 to 14.0.

- If the pH is *below* 7.0, then it is acidic.
- If the pH is *above* 7.0, then it is alkaline.
- If the pH is 7.0, then it is neutral.

The pH scale is logorhythmic. For us fishkeepers this becomes important because there is a tenfold difference between points on this scale. This means that water with a pH of 6.0 is *ten times* more acidic than water with a pH of 7.0. This same sample of water is *one hundred times* (ten times ten) more acidic than water with a pH of 8.0. This is one reason why it is so important to gradually adjust new fish to your water conditions.

pH is quite a simple parameter to measure, and there are plenty of commercially available test kits to do so. When you measure pH you are actually measuring the amount of free hydrogen ions ($H^+$) in a solution. If there are a great many, then it's acidic; if there are only few, it will be alkaline.

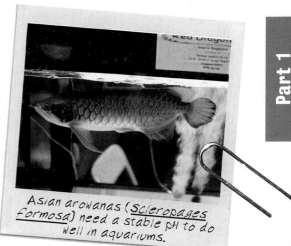

Asian arowanas (*Scleropages formosa*) need a stable pH to do well in aquariums.

The pH of a given body of water depends upon a variety of factors, particularly upon the underlying rocky strata, the surrounding environment (rain runoff can bring a lot of material into a lake or stream), and what falls into it, such as leaves and branches that can rot down and so lower the pH. In nature, then, freshwater fish are found in a wide range of pH. For example, freshwater fish are found in the waters of the Amazon, rich in humus and rotting vegetation, with pH's of 4.0 to 5.5. Freshwater fish are also found in the inland oceans of the Rift Valley lakes, such as Malawi and Tanganyika, with their extraor-dinarily high pH's of 7.8 to 8.5 and 8.7 to 9.4, respectively.

"Regular removal of biological waste material before it undergoes bacterial processing not only reduces the load on your filters but will also reduce the eventual nitrate levels. In brackish (and marine) aquaria, protein skimmers or refugiums are ideal, but even regular siphoning off of mulm will help in the short term."

If you are keeping wild-caught fish from such extreme habitats, then you may need to adjust the pH (as well as other

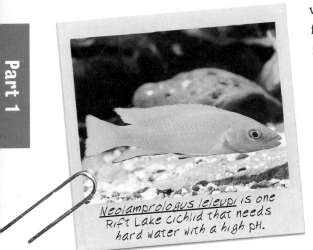

Neolamprologus leleupi is one Rift Lake Cichlid that needs hard water with a high pH.

water quality parameters) to suit these fish. Fortunately, the majority of freshwater fish available today are commercially bred and are much more tolerant of varying water conditions. Obvious examples include the neon tetra (*Paracheirodon innesi*) and discus (*Symphysodon* spp.), both bred around the world, particularly in Asia. Both of these species are endemics of Amazonian tributaries, yet modern strains cope well with typical tap water pH of over 7.0.

## Direct Effect

The fish's body goes to great lengths to control the pH level of its blood and other body fluids, because enzymes control most metabolic chemical reactions, and enzymes work best at certain pH levels. Drastic alterations in the pH of the surrounding water can exceed the ability of the body to maintain its pH within its necessary limits (usually around pH 7.4), which in turn can lead to serious internal complications. Low pH can induce an acidosis, while an excessively high pH can cause an alkalosis.

The signs of pH-related disease could be varied. Typically there is a marked escape response, with the fish hurtling around the aquarium or pond and even jumping above the surface. Mucus production is increased, and strands of mucus may be seen trailing from the skin and gills. If the pH is too low, it can affect the oxygen-carrying ability of the red blood cells, and so the fish may appear to gasp for air at the surface. The fins may fray and the skin may redden in patches. Eventually, if the fish is unable to adapt, it will gradually succumb and die.

In poorly managed aquaria there is often a gradual fall in pH over time, to which the long-term inhabitants may adjust with little or no apparent outward signs of problems. This fall in pH, together with other problems associated with poor care (such as high nitrate levels), can increase the susceptibility to disease, and the fish may just fail to thrive. New additions to the aquarium, on the other hand, will often die, showing signs consistent with sudden onset pH changes because they have no time to adjust. The following are some causes of low pH.

## Infrequent Water Changes

Over a period of time in ponds and aquaria there is a degree of buildup of acidic compounds such as carbonic acid from respiration and organic acids from metabolism. Biological filtration can also produce an increase in hydrogen ions due to bacterial metabolism. All of these can contribute to a slow but progressive fall in pH. This is easily remedied by undertaking regular water changes. Improving aeration or circulation may help to disperse more carbon dioxide.

## Poor Buffering Capacity

A buffer is a compound that protects against any temporary swings in pH. In aquaria the most important buffers are in the bicarbonate-carbonate system. Dissolved bicarbonate is usually in chemical equilibrium with carbonate, typically present as calcium carbonate found in calcareous rocks and gravel.

$$HCO_3^- \Longleftrightarrow H^+ + CO_3^{2-}$$

| $HCO_3^-$ | | $H^+$ | | $CO_3^{2-}$ |
|---|---|---|---|---|
| Bicarbonate ion | $\Longleftrightarrow$ | Hydrogen ion | + | Carbonate ion |
| | | | | (usually as calcium carbonate) |

With the above buffering system, if you add more acid ($H^+$) to the water, it will combine with spare carbonate ions to form bicarbonate ions, removing the extra $H^+$'s from solution and so preventing it from becoming more acidic. Carbonate ions can be recruited from calcium carbonate-containing materials if necessary.

Conversely, if there is a rise in pH due to a loss of hydrogen ions, more hydrogen ions are released from bicarbonate ions to counter this. As a result extra carbonate ions are formed. These are often deposited on surfaces as calcium carbonate crystals. Many high pH aquaria rely upon the use of buffering materials to help counteract the acidifying processes described above. Typically these are calcium carbonate-based and include such materials as tufa rock, coral sand, and oyster shells. These rely on compounds dissolving from them to counteract the increasing levels of hydrogen ions. Over time, the buffering capacity of such materials can become exhausted, and so regular changing of these materials is recommended (roughly every one to two years). Alternatively, specific buffering solutions are marketed for you to add to your pond or aquarium. The pH must be monitored closely and the instructions for these preparations followed to prevent pH crashes.

### *Acid Runoff*

Ponds surrounded by acidic soil may suffer low pH due to rain runoff bringing this material into the water. Improving local drainage and installation of small barriers may help to prevent this.

High levels of organic material such as leaves and branches will cause a progressive fall in pH, as bacterial and fungal degradation releases more organic acids into the water. In particular, ponds in temperate climates can suffer this problem, especially during the fall when huge numbers of shed leaves can be blown into the water. Placing mesh netting over your pond will catch many leaves, and seining with your net will help you to remove many others.

## Hardness

Hardness is a measure of the dissolved mineral content of a sample of water. Unfortunately, it is often confused with pH, but they are different. By far, the commonest mineral compound found in water is calcium carbonate, and so most methods that measure water hardness are designed to measure this compound. Water is not just a solution of calcium carbonate but also contains magnesium, bicarbonates, hydroxides, sulphides, chlorides, and even nitrates to name just a few. Trace elements are also present in varying concentrations. These include but are not limited to: zinc, iron, cobalt, iodine, and copper.

*Causes of Low pH*

During the night there is no photosynthesis going on, but the plants are still respiring— using oxygen and releasing carbon dioxide and so lowering the pH. This situation can lead to wide pH swings during the course of 24 hours and may severely stress any fish present.

There are several different units of measurement of general water hardness (GH), but fortunately they can all be converted into the standard measurement of *milligrams per liter* (mg/l) of calcium carbonate. Instead of mg/l, you may see it measured in *parts per million* (ppm). It's the same thing. These conversions are:

- 1° Hardness (USA) = 1.0mg/l calcium carbonate
- 1° Clark (UK) = 143mg/l calcium carbonate
- 1° dH (German) = 17.9mg/l calcium carbonate
- 1 milliequivalent (meq) = 50.0mg/l calcium carbonate

Historically, much of the advanced literature on fishkeeping has come out of either the United States or Germany, but even many of the American texts have adopted the German hardness scale. As a guide, the following table gives an idea of relative water hardness and the corresponding values.

MERTHYR TYDFIL PUBLIC LIBRARIES

## Carbonate Hardness (°KH)

This is a measurement of carbonate, bicarbonate, and hydroxide ions. These ions are involved with the main buffering systems and are able to neutralize acid. This is why the carbonate hardness is sometimes called the **alkalinity**. Therefore, the KH is the measure of the water's buffering capacity (i.e. its ability to neutralize acid). In the interests of simplicity, I will only use alkalinity to describe the pH, not the carbonate hardness.

## Non-carbonate Hardness (°NKH)

This is a measurement of those ions with little or no buffering activity, such as sulphates, chlorides, and nitrates.

## Temporary Hardness

This usually refers to bicarbonate levels. If you boil water, any bicarbonate comes out of solution as an insoluble carbonate precipitate, usually as calcium carbonate or magnesium carbonate.

## Permanent Hardness

This is the mineral content that is not removed by boiling. Salt (sodium chloride) does not directly affect hardness–it only makes water salty. Sea salts and rock salts do affect hardness because of other minerals associated with the salt.

## Conductivity

The electrical conductivity of a sample of water gives us an idea of the dissolved mineral levels (including salt) because the dissolved ions are needed to carry the current. Conductivity is measured in microsiemens ($\mu$ /cm), and a normal range would be around 180 to 480$\mu$.

As with pH, the hardness of natural waters is very variable, and this is reflected in the needs of our fish. High hardness waters typically have a high pH because of the high KH value. Using the same examples as for pH, Lake Malawi with a hardness of 200 to 220mg/l of calcium carbonate (12° to 13°dH) and Lake Tanganyika at 200 to 240mg/l calcium carbonate (12° to 14°dH). At the other extreme, although the tributaries that coalesce to form the main the main Amazon are divided into three types of water (blackwater, clear water, and white water) depending upon their appearance, all of these waters have minimal hardnesses, occasionally below 18mg/l (1°dH). It is likely that volume here gives water conditions some stability; maintaining an aquarium at these levels is very difficult and fraught with problems.

The importance of hardness to fish largely has to do with osmoregulation. Consider that in a freshwater fish, all of the salts, proteins, and so on inside it mean that its body fluids are more concentrated than the surrounding water. The fish is "leaky" to small molecules such as water. Large molecules like proteins cannot normally be lost from the body, but there are microscopic gaps between cells that will allow water molecules to pass through them.

In this situation, water will pass from a more dilute solution (the water outside of the fish) into a more concentrated solution (fluids inside the fish) through these tiny gaps in an effort to dilute the fish's body fluids down to the same level as that of the surrounding water. This process is known as **osmosis**.

Fishes osmoregulate, and freshwater fish keep their body fluids at the correct concentration by either eliminating excess water as urine or by controlling their salt levels by balancing salt loss in urine with intake either from food or from the surrounding water.

In softer water there is a greater difference between the concentration of the fish's body fluid and the surrounding water, so more water enters the fish and then needs to be eliminated. This takes extra energy. In harder water, less energy is utilized to do this because less water enters and so there is less osmotic stress on the fish.

Fish have evolved to suit their own localized environment. Fish from soft waters will not only have kidneys adapted to eliminating larger quantities of water, but also their guts and gills will be designed to extract maximum amounts of important ions such as calcium out of the water. Placing such fish in hard water may bring about a mineral overload, stretching the kidney's abilities to eliminate these extra ions out of the body. In such fish calcium deposits may form in the kidneys. Hardwater fish placed in soft water will have to do the opposite, increasing their scavenging of necessary ions above their normal levels and expelling increased volumes of urine. In both cases extra physiological stress is placed on the fish. Fish can adapt to altered water constitution, providing that they are allowed sufficient time and the differences do not exceed their physiologic capability.

In very soft water, low calcium concentrations can result in poor bone formation and increased disease susceptibility. For soft water species, hard water can reduce egg viability. This is because egg hardening is secondary to ions absorbed by osmosis. If the water is quite hard, then fewer ions will be taken across the egg membrane. Increasing KH will increase the alkalinity and can potentiate ammonia toxicity.

## Correcting Water Hardness

If the hardness is too high, then dilution with very soft water is needed. Soft water is usually obtained by:

• **Reverse Osmosis**–Forcing tap water across a selectively permeable membrane that only allows water molecules through makes R.O. water. Water obtained this way is virtually pure.

• **Ion Exchange Resins**–Use only those designed for aquarium use, not for domestic use. Household ion exchangers (so-called water softeners) swap calcium ions for sodium ions. This does lower the hardness, but the abnormally high sodium levels can lead to serious problems.

• **Rainwater Dilution**–In theory this is a good, ecologically sound way to soften water. In practice, you must make sure that the water collected does not become contaminated with pollution.

• **Peat Filtration**–Use aquarium peat, not gardening peat. It softens water by exchanging calcium ions for hydrogen ions. Resultant water is soft and acidic and usually contains significant amounts of tannins that stain the water a pale tea-like color. For those of you with an environmental conscience, it may be better to avoid the use of peat to reduce the pressure on peat bogs around the world.

| General Hardness (mg/l calcium carbonate) | General Hardness (°dH) | Water Hardness Rating |
|---|---|---|
| 0 – 50 | 0 –3 | Very Soft |
| 50 – 100 | 3 –6 | Moderately Soft |
| 100 – 150 | 6 – 9 | Slightly Hard |
| 150 – 200 | 9 – 12 | Moderately Hard |
| 200 – 300 | 12 – 18 | Hard |
| 300 + | 18+ | Very Hard |

If the water hardness is too soft, it can be corrected by the addition of calcium carbonate-containing materials, such as coral sand, tufa rock, dolomite, or oyster shells. Commercial aquarium buffers are available from your local aquarium supply shops that will increase the GH and KH. Specific salt preparations, such as Rift Valley mixes, are also available to add to water to mimic the hardness and pH of these habitats.

## Oxygen

Oxygen constitutes 20% of atmospheric air, but because it's relatively insoluble in water, there is 20 to 30 times less oxygen in a given volume of water than in an equivalent volume of air. Almost all of the oxygen dissolved in water gets there by dissolving into it at the surface. Recommended levels of oxygen are above 6.0mg/l at 25°C for freshwater tropical fish and 8.0mg/l (with a minimum of 5.0mg/l) for pond fish.

If dissolved oxygen levels fall too low, the fish will start to gasp at the surface. They will often congregate around filter outlets and other areas of increased water turbulence, as these create localized areas of higher oxygenation. Breathing rates increase and the gill covers will be pumping harder and faster. Unfortunately, this increase in muscle activity will actually *increase* the fishes' oxygen requirements. Fish seen mouthing at the surface are not usually "gasping for air" but are trying to draw the thin surface film of oxygenated water across their gills; unless they have special respiratory structures, most fish cannot utilize atmospheric oxygen. If this does not improve matters, the fish will become comatose and die. Fish that have died in this way have flared operculae, wide-open mouths, and pale gills. Larger fish with greater body weights have disproportionately higher oxygen demands, and it is these fish that show overt signs (and in the worst cases, die) first.

Many fish naturally come from waters that are seasonally or permanently low in oxygen and so have alternative strategies of surviving. Fish groups such as the anabantids have a special organ, called the labyrinth, which has evolved partly from the gills and allows them to breathe atmospheric air. Corydoras catfish and loaches use the lining of their intestines to absorb air swallowed from the surface, while in lungfish (*Protopterus* and *Lepidosiren*) the swim bladder has evolved into distinct lung-like structures. Some fish deal with low oxygen levels in a different fashion, by developing metabolic pathways that function without oxygen. Goldfish, Crucian carp (*Carassius carassius*), and koi are three species that switch to anaerobic pathways in times of low oxygen. However, prolonged exposure to these conditions can risk an acidosis of their tissues secondary to lactic acid buildup.

### Low dissolved oxygen levels can occur because of:

• **High stocking densities**—Obviously, the more fish there are, the more oxygen is consumed. Remember that plants in the same system also use oxygen throughout the day and night, and it is only during the hours of daylight that they produce more by photosynthesis than they use. The bacteria in the biological filters are also constantly consuming large volumes of oxygen. Large amounts of decaying material can reduce the available dissolved oxygen content.

• **High temperatures**—The warmer the water is (to a point) the less dissolved oxygen it can hold. Therefore, even if you maintain warmwater species, be sure to always provide adequate aeration in the form of air bubbles or any other method that will result in surface agitation.

• **Salinity**—Salt water holds less oxygen than freshwater, a fact that must be considered not just with marine aquaria but with brackish water collections and hospital aquaria with high salt levels.

• **Altitude**—Higher altitudes reduce oxygen levels. This rarely becomes a consideration.

• **Low atmospheric pressure**—Sudden fish deaths in ponds have been associated with periods of stormy weather when low atmospheric pressure, often accompanied by high temperatures, triggers a fall in dissolved oxygen.

In times of high environmental temperatures such as heat waves or air-conditioning breakdown, one can attempt to lower the temperature of aquaria by floating plastic bags containing ice in the tanks. Do not just place ice into aquaria, as the melting water may alter the water chemistry or introduce problem chemicals such as chlorine.

In some instances there is an excess of dissolved oxygen in the water, resulting in a supersaturation. This can result in a condition known as gas bubble disease, where obvious gas bubbles can be seen in the fins, skin and occasionally behind the eye.

Oxygen is not very soluble in water. In oxygen supersaturated water, any event which causes a decrease in the partial pressure of the dissolved oxygen will cause oxygen to come out of solution. This oxygen will form itself into obvious bubbles in the blood vessels, especially those of the fins, skin, and occasionally behind the eye. Fins become frayed and hemorrhagic. If the swim bladder is involved, the fish may lose its ability to balance. Fortunately, the fish usually come to no lasting harm, and the condition sorts itself out once the surrounding water loses enough oxygen to be no longer supersaturated.

## Carbon Dioxide

Carbon dioxide is a byproduct of aerobic respiration and is released by not only fish and plants, but by bacteria as well. It is, however, also utilized by plants for photosynthesis.

*Management of Carbon Dioxide Levels*

- Reduce stocking densities
- Control plant or algal growth
- Improve circulation or aeration

Unlike oxygen, it is highly soluble in water, where it forms carbonic acid; however, just as with ammonia, the dissolved carbon dioxide is in equilibrium with carbonic acid and the bicarbonate ion. This is represented below:

$$CO_2 \quad + \quad H_2O \iff H_2CO_3 \iff HCO_3^- \; + \; H^+.$$

carbon dioxide  +  carbonic    bicarbonate ion    hydrogen ion
water           acid

Note that at the other end of the equations is a free hydrogen ion. This is why carbon dioxide has such an effect on the pH of water. Carbon dioxide produced from respiration is exhaled from the gills. If there are high levels of carbon dioxide in the water, then the pH will fall. This also reduces the ability of the fish to remove carbon dioxide from its body, and so the tissues of the fish become too acidic. This is what is known as an acidosis, and it affects a wide range of normal body fluids.

In extreme cases, an anesthetic-like narcosis develops, and the fish will become very sluggish and may die. Prolonged exposure to carbon dioxide levels greater than 10 to 20mg/l has been linked to nephrocalcinosis, a condition where mineral deposits form in the kidney.

## Chlorine

Chlorine, or its ammonium compound chloramine, is added to domestic supplies by water companies to help sterilize our tap water. Dissolved chlorine forms hypochlorous acid and hypochlorite. The concentrations of these two are pH and temperature dependant. Hypochlorous acid is the more toxic compound of the two and is favored by lower temperatures and a pH of less than 7.5. Chlorine does not remain stable in water, so water companies calculate the dosage so there is still an active concentration at the farthest point down the line (your tap).

Chloramine is more stable, and it also has the toxicity problems associated with ammonia as well as chlorine. Chlorine damages cell membranes and enzymes, and even levels of 4.0ppm have been known to cause mortalities in goldfish and koi within eight hours of exposure. If fish are constantly exposed to low levels, such as 0.2 to 0.3ppm (levels often found in tap water), deaths can occur after around three weeks. Long-term exposure to levels as low as 0.002ppm can induce gill hyperplasia (thickening), affecting the fish's ability to take in oxygen.

With sudden exposure, fish show an escape reaction. They may become discolored, with reddened patches and areas of damage (often referred to as burns) on the fins, gills, and skin. The fish eventually appear weakened and die of respiratory failure due to gill damage. Extremely high levels can cause sudden deaths with no obvious clinical signs.

### Dealing With Chlorine

Because chlorine is so unstable, aerating water well before using it in water changes, or leaving it to stand for 24 hours should dissipate most of the chlorine.

Commercial tap water conditioners are available that contain sodium thiosulphate that will actively bind any chlorine present. Zeolite can be used to absorb any ammonia if chloramine is used.

## Environmental Toxins

There is a wide range of poisonous chemicals that can cause havoc in ponds and aquaria. The list is long and would include such obvious chemicals as garden pesticides and herbicides, certain pet flea control products (particularly organophosphate sprays and pyrethroids), and cigarette smoke. One particular danger is from heavy metal poisoning and can be due to exposure to metallic objects, such as coins and pipe work. Metals known to cause problems are lead, copper, iron, zinc cadmium, and aluminum.

Heavy metal toxicity depends upon the pH and temperature. The lower the pH and the higher the temperature, the more soluble these metals become. As an example, at pH values higher than 7.0, iron precipitates out as iron hydroxide, coating the gills and causing severe breathing problems and even death. Aluminum is toxic at pH levels over 8.0.

It is very difficult to give accurate toxicity levels for heavy metals because both water hardness and chemical reactions with other dissolved substances can have a significant effect on how toxic it is. Also, many dangerous effects are due to long-term or cumulative exposure, and so testing of water levels and setting "safe" parameters may be of limited value.

Long-term exposure to damaging levels can lead to disease in the gills, kidneys, and liver, which in turn can lead to osmotic imbalance, respiratory problems, poor growth rates, deformities, and breeding difficulties. Hatching fry may have deformities.

Long-term heavy metal poisoning can lead to immune suppression, increasing susceptibility to secondary infections. This is particularly so with copper and to a lesser extent, aluminum. Prolonged exposure to toxic levels of cadmium, mercury, lead, and zinc has been associated with anemia. Sudden exposures to high levels can cause large-scale losses, especially of younger fish. Sudden death in fish transferred into galvanized containers has been linked to zinc poisoning.

## Electricity

Modern fishkeeping involves the use of a variety of electrical equipment. The risk of faulty equipment holds inherent dangers not only for the aquarist but also for the fish. Spinal deformations and vertebral fractures have been linked to electrocution in fish. It is thought that this is due to severe contraction of the muscles along the back, particularly beneath the dorsal fin where the muscle mass is greatest.

Due to the high risk associated with electrical products, it is suggested that you call a certified electrician should you need to have special alterations done on your aquarium. Certified electricians are highly trained and often work with special aquarium installation projects. If you are unsure about which electrician is best for your needs, consult a local aquarium retailer or aquarium maintenance company for their recommendations.

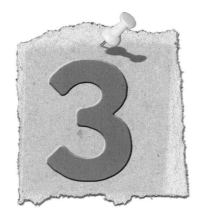

# An Approach to Disease

Infectious diseases are what most fishkeepers are concerned with when they worry about fish diseases in general. Some of these, such as white spot disease caused by *Ichthyophthirius multifiliis*, occur very commonly. Once detected, any fishkeeper should be able to recognize it in its usual presentation. Other infectious diseases may be seen less often but are no less important.

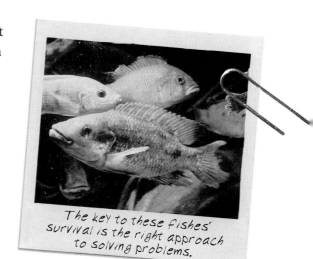

The key to these fishes' survival is the right approach to solving problems.

*Arriving at a Diagnosis Involves the Following Steps:*

- Reviewing how the fish is being kept.
- Making an accurate examination and description of what is wrong with the fish.
- Performing any further tests that can reasonably be done.
- Adding all of the information from steps 1 to 3 and comparing the information with the disease descriptions contained in this book.

Selecting an appropriate treatment involves arriving at a correct diagnosis, or to put it another way, if your diagnosis is wrong, then your treatment will not likely work. Health professionals (such as veterinarians) do have access to other people and facilities, such as commercial laboratories, which are able to offer specialist services like bacterial culture or electron microscopy to achieve a definitive diagnosis. Such backup is not usually available to the hobbyist, but fortunately there are steps that the hobbyist can follow to go a long way toward diagnosing fish disease in the pond or aquarium. One can also attempt treatment with one of the variety of proprietary medications. It is, however, an unfortunate fact that many of these off-the-shelf preparations are of limited value at best, but that will be discussed later.

There is an immediate temptation to focus your attention on the problems of an individual sick fish and thereby completely miss the bigger

*Essential points to look at are:*

- Species you are dealing with
- Stocking density
- Companion species
- Ammonia levels
- Nitrite levels
- Nitrate levels
- pH
- Temperature

picture. If I have a koi with an ulcer, then in all probability it will be due to a bacterial infection. I can treat for this, but if I do not step back and realize that the stocking density of the pond is around 50% too high, and as a result the

*Other points to consider are:*

- Hardness and KH
- Are there quarantine facilities?
- Food offered
- Lighting
- Use of accessory oxygenation devices
- Exposure to metallic objects

nitrite reading is consistently around 1.0mg/l, then the koi will not improve. This koi has an infection because high nitrite levels compromise its immune system, which in turn is a result of overstocking–ALWAYS look at the bigger picture!

## Performing An Accurate Examination

We are now going to look at the behavior and the physical condition of the fish. To do this accurately you need to be familiar with the species or variety of fish that you are dealing with, but there are certain general points that you can use.

Foremost, a healthy fish is generally an alert fish. Most aquarium and pond fish respond to what is happening both in and out of the water. They react to each other and will commonly acknowledge the presence of their owner by begging for food. Opening the aquarium lid or standing by the pond will, in the majority of cases, elicit a crowding at the surface of open mouths. Be aware of the fish that does not do this, especially if it is normally a glutton.

This is where your knowledge of different fish species comes in useful, because some fish are not, by nature, bright and bold. They naturally hide, displaying both cryptic coloration and behavior either to avoid predation

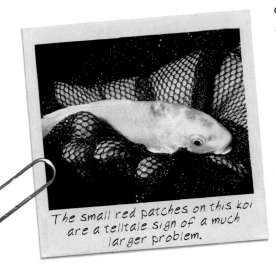

The small red patches on this koi are a telltale sign of a much larger problem.

or as a means of stalking prey. An example of the use of this cryptic coloration would be with the South American leaf-fish (*Monocirrhus polyacanthus*) and loricarid catfish (*Farlowella acus*). The African freshwater pipefish (*Enneacanthus ansorgii*) arguably does both.

Healthy fish normally put on a show. Fins are erect when the fish comes to a standstill, and their colors are clear and distinct, if not necessarily bright (depending upon the species). Fish live in a fish-eat-fish world, and so a good survival tactic is to advertise your health. This behavior is instinctive because most predators are looking for an easy catch. If you show you are fit and healthy, then you may be overlooked in preference for a slower, sicker fish. This is a double-edged sword for us fishkeepers because occasionally we can be caught out of water–the behavior to put on a show is instinctive, so even sick fish will attempt to do this. It is often only once a fish is too ill to have the energy to pretend to be well that it begins to show signs of illness.

## Common Physical Signs of a Sick Fish

A dulling of the skin color or a patchy appearance can be due to a thickening of the mucous cover on the scales. In some cases, the mucus may hang off the fish in threads, where it may be mistaken as a fungal infection. This is commonly seen with external parasitic infestations or water-quality problems. Torn fins heal readily, but reddening and blood streaking suggest a bacterial infection may be established. Fins that are permanently clamped and appear thickened are also signs of ill health.

The skin should appear smooth, and scales, where present, should be well defined and regular. Scales sit in the deeper levels of the skin (the dermis), and so the loss of a scale can be a deep breach in the skin and may allow a secondary infection by bacteria or fungi to take root. Bloody or reddened patches are of concern, while ulceration is very serious.

Erratic swimming may indicate a rapid deterioration in water quality. Bumping into the sides and objects in the aquarium may be due to a central nervous system problem (including blindness), as may spiral and circling motions through the water column as well. In mollies and other livebearers, shimmying—the rapid, exaggerated sideways swimming movements that take the fish nowhere—is a sign of a flavobacterial infection. These bacteria release toxins that affect the fish's brain, thus triggering such abnormal behavior.

A loss of body mass (wasting disease) can be due to a failure to feed properly, underfeeding, internal parasites, and some infections such as mycobacteriosis. A swelling of the body can be seen with internal tumors, egg retention, large burdens of parasitic worms, and fluid accumulation due to kidney and other major organ disease.

Changes in normal behavior, such as skulking, hiding, reduced or loss of appetite, abnormal swimming patterns, or any obvious deviation from the fish's normal swimming pattern, should be a cause for concern.

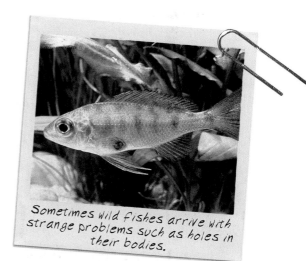

Sometimes wild fishes arrive with strange problems such as holes in their bodies.

Some altered behavior can be very specific. For example, fish mouthing at the surface or hanging around areas of high water turbulence, such as filter outlets, are likely to be striving to increase their oxygen intake. If you observed this, you would consider gill disease, low dissolved oxygen content, or malachite green toxicity as major possibilities.

Blood-red patches or streaks that look like bruising, ulcers, cotton wool-like fungal growths, and large mobile parasites such as fish lice (*Argulus*) are all obvious maladies that can be seen with the naked eye.

What tests can you, the hobbyist, do to help arrive at a diagnosis? Water-quality tests are of tremendous value and should always be done; if necessary, they should be repeated on a regular basis. Other tests, such as skin scrapes, require a degree of skill and practical experience plus some relatively expensive equipment like a light microscope. If you feel that it is necessary to go down this line, it may be better for you to consider seeking the services of a veterinarian, but make inquiries first. It is a sad fact that not all members of my profession share both the interest and skill in dealing with fish that they may have with your cat or horse. Those who do, however, are often worth every cent of their fee.

By comparing all of the information in this chapter to the disease descriptions contained later in this book, you should arrive at an accurate diagnosis. In some cases, it should at least take you into the correct area, which may be all that is necessary.

# Part Two
# A Closer Look at Common Fish Diseases

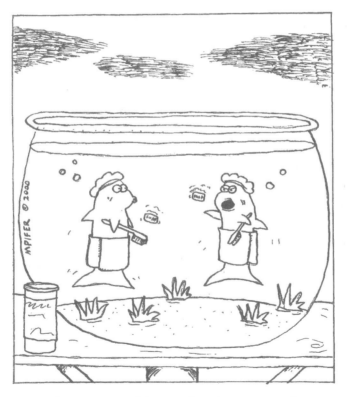

*"Francis, who are we kidding? There's no way we're going to get clean in this place! We're just soaking in our own filth!"*

# Viral Disease

Viruses are the smallest structures known that are also able to replicate themselves. In some cases, they are so small that they need to hijack some of their host's DNA in order to replicate. Treatment of viral disease is very much in its infancy, and in general viruses cannot be medicated. Treatment is usually supportive by providing good food and water quality to give the fish its best chance of fending off

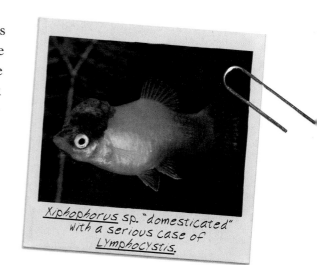

*Xiphophorus* sp. "domesticated" with a serious case of Lymphocystis.

the infection itself. Just as with humans and the common cold, aspirins and paracetamols may make us feel better. However, we rely upon our immune systems to remove the infection from our bodies.

## Lymphocystis

A particular type of virus known as an iridovirus causes *Lymphocystis* disease. This virus can live for many days freely in the water, and fishes may become infected through cuts, abrasions, or by eating infected material. *Lymphocystis* virus invades individual cells and triggers a massive enlargement of that cell, often up to 500 times its original size. This enlargement is often so extreme that these cells can be easily seen with the naked eye. They appear as whitish or grayish nodules that can be several millimeters in diameter. Some of these nodules have a good blood supply, and obvious blood vessels may be seen, which give these nodules a pinkish appearance. Unfortunately, nodules can also occur internally and can act as space-occupying lesions, compressing and affecting those organs around them.

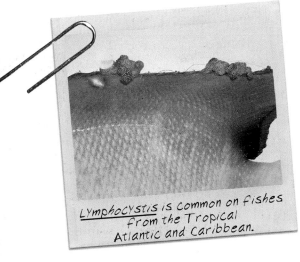

Lymphocystis is common on fishes from the Tropical Atlantic and Caribbean.

In the face of infection, the affected fish will commonly mount an inflammatory response, and eventually the fish will eliminate the virus from its system. It would appear that immunity is usually solid, as recurrence is rare in healthy fish. The duration of this whole process can be from several weeks to several months.

Any trauma that allows infective viral particles to gain access to damaged tissue provides a possible means of infection. A celebrated case was the linking of this viral infection with "colored" glassfish *Chanda ranga*, where it seemed that these fish were becoming infected following the injection of the colored dyes. It would seem that transmission between species of the same genus is easier than across species barriers, leading to the suggestion that there are many different species or genus-specific strains. Stress will

> "Most freshwater fishes appear to be susceptible, but members of the cyprinid (carp-like) family do not become infected."

increase susceptibility to this infection–it is not uncommon to see it in newly imported fishes, for instance.

## What to Look For

The large growths seen are typical of this infection. Occasional reddening due to hemorrhages is occasionally noted when these growths are accidentally traumatized.

Microscopic examination is usually unnecessary for diagnosis, but on a squash preparation of a tissue sample, clusters of the hugely enlarged individual cells can be observed. Each affected cell appears as an obvious circular structure.

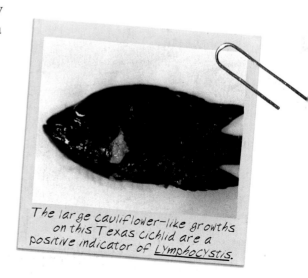

The large cauliflower-like growths on this Texas cichlid are a positive indicator of _Lymphocystis_.

This disease is usually self-limiting. Fish appear to be able to mount a good immune response, and with good care and nutrition, the growths will spontaneously disappear. Be patient–do not be

**Part 2**

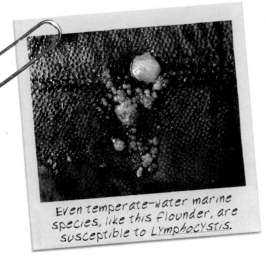

Even temperate-water marine species, like this flounder, are susceptible to Lymphocystis.

tempted to cut or otherwise remove the growths because doing so is likely to trigger even more growths at that site.

*Lymphocystis* is very characteristic in appearance, but it could possibly be mistaken for tumors. Another possibility is epitheliocystis, which is a disease caused by a very different, bacterial-like organism that infects the mucous-secreting cells of the skin and gills. Epitheliocystis is well recognized in cyprinids, such as carp; if *Lymphocystis*-like masses are seen on these fish, then treat for epitheliocystis!

You can control *Lymphocystis* by keeping your fish in the best of health to help them resist infection and eliminate it as quickly as possible should it occur. Quarantine all new stock for at least four weeks. Ultraviolet sterilization may reduce the risk of waterborne transmission.

## Other Iridoviral Diseases

Iridoviruses have been documented as causing high mortalities in cichlids such as angelfish (*Pterophyllum* spp.) and Ramirez's dwarf cichlid (*Mikrogeophagus ramirezi*); anabantids including three spot gouramis (*Trichogaster trichopterus*) and dwarf gouramis (*Colisa lalia*); and the lampeye killifish (*Aplocheilichthys normani*). Infected three spot gouramis became lethargic and show darkened coloration; in some, the abdomen appears enlarged due to an accumulation of fluid, and the spleen may swell. Up to 50% can die within 24 to 48 hours. In orange chromides (*Etroplus maculatus*), an iridovirus has been linked to anemia; infected fish were thin and pale, and the gills and internal organs were generally very pale due to the anemia.

Part 2

## Spring Viraemia of Carp (SVC)

SVC is caused by a rhabdovirus (a group of viruses that also includes rabies). It is sometimes known as *Rhabdovirus carpio.*

Infected fish shed the virus into the surrounding water in their feces, often in mucous anal casts. Other fish then inhale viral particles suspended in the water, where they attach to the gills. Here they invade and replicate before spreading throughout the blood stream to infect the internal organs. Incubation time for SVC varies from 7 to 60 days, depending upon water temperature.

A classic case of SVC occurs when the virus damages and so causes inflammation of the lining of blood vessels. This in turn makes them "leaky," allowing both fluid and red blood cells to leak out into the surrounding tissues. This means that SVC causes hemorrhages and edema (fluid buildup) in a number of tissues, including the heart, brain, and intestines. In the kidneys there is serious damage to the microscopic tubes, affecting their ability to function properly. Pancreatic tissue is often very inflamed.

With classic SVC, infected fish may show a buildup of fluid in the abdominal cavity, which is suggestive of "dropsy." In this case, fluid accumulates in the body cavity, making the fish appear swollen–this pressure can build up so much that the anus may be partially forced out and prolapsed. The eyes may even bulge (exophthalmia) due to fluid in the eye sockets. Those tissues involved with the immune response, such as the spleen and the cranial kidney, often show marked reactive changes. Further changes that are often described are thought by many to be due to secondary bacterial infection and would include ulceration and accumulations of pus-like material inside the body cavity.

**Part 2**

## Swim Bladder Inflammation (SBI)

In this form, only the swim bladder is targeted. Marked hemorrhages occur on the swim bladder surface, and there is serious damage to its lining. Such fish lose their balance and coordination before eventually dying. This disease is said to be due to a second rhabdovirus called SBI (Swim Bladder Inflammation) virus, although it is as yet impossible to distinguish it from the SVC virus.

In both cases there are often mass mortalities that can continue for weeks. Low or rapidly fluctuating temperatures can predispose fish to infection if the virus is present. Infected fish produce interferon as part of their antiviral response, but unfortunately, interferon production is temperature dependant. This means that above a temperature of 68°F, immunity is usually quite good. At 52° to 68°F, obvious clinical signs occur, but some fish are able to mount an immune response and survive. At temperatures below 50°F, the fish immune response is so sluggish that viral multiplication (which is itself reduced by the low temperatures) is able to continue unchecked, causing mortalities.

Fish lice (*Argulus*) and leeches (*Piscicola*) have been implicated with transmission of SVC from fish to fish, as have herons in transferring virus between ponds. Contaminated equipment may also help to spread infection.

### What to Look For

This disease is virtually confined to members of the carp family. Many cyprinid fish, apart from koi and common carp, can be affected, including goldfish, grass carp, and tench. The picture is further complicated by the fact that some infected fish may harbor the virus but not show clinical signs. I have seen one case where only koi became ill and died–goldfish and rudd in the same pond were not clinically affected. Some non-cyprinids, such as pike (*Esox* spp.) and Wels catfish (*Siluris glanis*), can also become infected.

Affected fish will often show a darkened body color. Hemorrhages can be present both internally and externally. The anus may become partially prolapsed and may be observed bulging out. Infected fish are weak, breathe shallowly, and may have a thick, mucoid cast trailing from the anus. Gills are often pale.

If SVC presents itself as a swim bladder inflammation, infected fish will lose their balance and

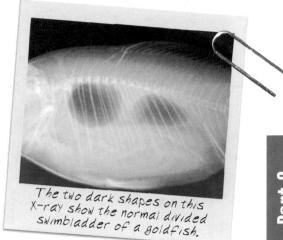

The two dark shapes on this X-ray show the normal divided swimbladder of a goldfish.

will be seen lying on their side at the bottom or floating beneath the surface. If the fish swim, their movements are wobbly and uncoordinated. Usually no hemorrhages can be seen. A definitive diagnosis can really be done only by a professional laboratory and involves isolating virus from infected tissue.

There is as yet no effective treatment for SVC. In theory, supportive management would be appropriate. This would include antibiotics to prevent secondary infections and adding salt to the water to help with osmoregulation, but most fish exhibiting signs of the disease will die, especially at low temperatures.

In the United Kingdom, SVC is a notifiable disease under the Diseases of the Fish Act 1937. This means that if it is strongly suspected or diagnosed, it must be reported to DEFRA. Testing is carried out at the CEFAS laboratories at Weymouth. If SVC is found, then the owner of the infected fish has two choices:

Part 2

• Euthanasia of all in-contact potentially susceptible fish, followed by disinfection of the pond, equipment, etc. This is carried out by DEFRA personnel.

• Becoming a designated infected zone. In practice, this means no fish are allowed in or out for a period of three years, with the lifting of this restriction only after a designated period when tests have proved consistently negative for SVC.

A similar situation exists in the United States. Any suspected SVC cases must be reported to the USDA (United States Department of Agriculture). Suspected cases may be quarantined or destroyed in line with the situation in the United Kingdom. Classic SVC can closely mimic a bacterial septicemia or a severe parasitic infestation. The ubiquitous presence of *Aeromonas* bacteria in pond water and on fish wounds can easily mislead one into making a diagnosis of bacterial disease. Mass mortalities, especially if largely affecting koi, carp, or other susceptible species that fail to respond to usual antibacterial medications, should be considered suspect particularly if weather/temperature conditions have been suitable for this virus. The presence of severe gill lesions in koi with Koi Herpes Virus should allow its distinction from SVC in cases of multiple deaths.

There is no way of preventing the disease other than quarantining all new stock. Vaccination has been tried and appears to be reasonably effective at temperatures above 68°F, but these are unlikely to be made available in countries where SVC is notifiable, as vaccination may interfere by masking disease outbreaks.

## Cichlid Rhabdovirus

This virus is also known as Rio Grande perch rhabdovirus (RGPR). Originally discovered as a cause of lethargy and death in the Texas cichlid (*H. cyanoguttatum,* also known as the Rio Grande perch), this infection also caused 80% losses in convict cichlids (*Cryptoheros nigrofasciatum*) and *Tilapia zilli.*

## Carp Pox

Carp pox is actually caused by a typical alpha-herpes virus, and it is probably better called cyprinid herpes virus-1 (CHV-1). CHV-1 causes groups of skin cells to proliferate into small masses or growths. These growths, known as papillomas, are often whitish or grayish and resemble blobs of candle wax. They can occur anywhere on the body but particularly affect the mouth area, head and upper surface, and the fins. Experimental exposure of carp to CHV-1 revealed that these growths appeared five to six months after infection. After a period of time, the growths are shed and disappear, with no apparent trace that they ever existed. But don't be fooled–unfortunately, a large percentage of infected fish do not eliminate the virus from their body; instead, it "hides" from the immune system in certain cells of the body, including the cranial nerves, spinal nerves, and some skin tissues.

Such infected fish are highly likely to remain infected for the rest of their lives, with recurrences of the infection and hence reappearances of the papillomas usually occurring around seven to eight months after their disappearance. In the pond situation, CHV-1 recurrence occurs most often in late fall, with the number of growths and the number of fish showing signs increasing over the winter and into the spring.

If you are wondering why this happens, think of cold sores! If you suffer from cold sores (a human herpes virus), it will often show itself when you are unwell. When you are unwell or run down, your body is less able to fend off infections because your immune system is suppressed. The same happens with koi in cold weather. As temperatures drop, their immune systems do not work so well and the virus is able to multiply and express itself. With the arrival of spring the CHV-1 growths shrink and fall off, because as the weather improves and temperatures increase, the fish are better able to mount an effective immune response, thereby stopping viral production and shedding the wax-like papillomas.

Generally, for most healthy adult koi, CHV-1 represents a nuisance condition. It temporarily disfigures the individual but is of no consequence. In young carp it can be fatal, and it has been linked to skull abnormalities. In other cases, CHV-1 has been suggested as a trigger for the formation of malignant tumors in carp, especially squamous cell carcinomas. These are invasive skin tumors that are often found around the mouth and may require surgery or possibly chemotherapy to control.

High stocking densities will help the virus to spread, as will anything that damages the protective integrity of the skin and mucous covering, such as ectoparasites (especially *Argulus* spp.) and trauma or abrasions.

## What to Look For

This virus is usually seen only in the varieties of cultured carp (*Cyprinus carpio*), such as mirror carp, leather carp, and koi. It can infect other cyprinids such as Crucian carp and grass carp but is rarely fatal, even in the young of these species. This virus triggers wax-like growths on the skin and fins. In those cases where the virus triggers tumors to form, then these may appear as rough, wart-like masses often around the mouth but potentially anywhere on the body surface. Heavy losses may be encountered in young fry.

There is no effective treatment. This condition is usually self-limiting and will disappear, albeit temporarily. Recurrence is common, most often when temperatures drop again in the fall, although it can occur when the fish become stressed by other causes. Treatment with anti-herpes drugs such as acyclovir has been suggested, but it is of doubtful use and usually unnecessary.

CHV-1 could be mistaken for other causes of firm swellings such as fibromas, granuloma (areas of thickened inflammation), and epitheliocystis. This last disease is infectious and is caused by the bacteria-like organism chlamydia. It triggers whitish growths to occur not unlike *Lymphocystis*, an iridovirus.

Strict quarantine of all newly bought stock will stop the introduction of this virus into established collections. If you don't want it in your collection, don't buy from ponds or vats where there are fish showing typical pox growths. In particular, this applies to those retailers that keep their larger koi for sale in ponds along with some resident fish; if these permanent fish are infected, they will continually infect any new, non-infected koi that are brought in by the retailer.

## Koi Herpes Virus (KHV)

Koi herpes virus (KHV) is a relatively new disease that has been causing great anguish and consternation around the world. It appears to be specific for koi and other carp (*Cyprinus carpio*) varieties. Even closely related cyprinids such as goldfish (*Carassius auratus*) do not appear to become clinically ill when exposed to the virus. This disease has been

*Main Predisposing Factors to an Outbreak of KHV*

**Temperature**—Mortalities up to 95% can occur within the permissive temperature range of 64° to 77°F

**Stress**—Overcrowding and particularly the movement of fishes from one aquarium or pond to another are likely to trigger outbreaks.

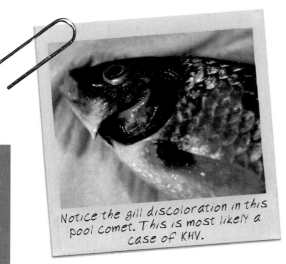

Notice the gill discoloration in this pool Comet. This is most likely a case of KHV.

detected worldwide, with outbreaks recorded in Israel, Japan, Asia, the United States, and the United Kingdom.

The best that one can say at present is that KHV is a herpes-like virus. It appears to be very similar to herpes viruses in some respects, but it is sufficiently different enough to have an alternative name suggested. This is carp nephritis and gill necrosis virus (CNGV), a name that reflects the damage this virus causes.

It seems highly likely that infection occurs through the gills. If the water temperature is between 68° to 79°F, then the virus causes extensive damage to the gills. Infection of koi with KHV at a water temperature of 73°F ended with a total mortality of 95%. The disease progressed rapidly at 82°F, but there was a marginally lower mortality of around 89% to 95%. At 62°F the death rate was 85%, but no deaths occurred at 55°F. However, moving these virus-exposed fish from 55° to 72°F triggered a rapid onset of the disease and subsequent deaths.

KHV-infected fish show obvious gill discoloration and necrosis (dying off) of infected gill tissue. This may appear in distinct patches with loss of tissue down to the cartilage of the primary lamellae. Secondary bacterial and fungal infections readily establish themselves. The fish appear to lose much of their mucous coat, they appear thin, and the eyes are often sunken in appearance. This may be due to a combination of oxygen starvation from the gill damage and the damage to the kidneys seen in many individuals.

## What to Look For

Only koi and other varieties of carp (*Cyprinus carpio*) are affected. Goldfish and other cyprinids will not be showing any signs of disease. In a full-blown outbreak, many koi and other carp will be seen dead and dying. The water temperature will be in the permissive range of 68° to 76°F. Infected fish will appear lethargic and will swim close to the water surface.

Severe gill damage will lead them to gather in areas with high oxygen levels, such as water inlets or waterfalls. There will be obvious respiratory distress (increased breathing rate, gasping at surface). In coordination (fishes bumping into objects) such as that resulting from a swim bladder inflammation may also result, especially in severe cases. The skin and gills will exhibit a decreased mucus production, and furthermore, there may be hemorrhages in fins and in the body. Examination under the operculae (gill covers) will reveal severe gill necrosis. This appears as white, gray, or black, and damage and erosion to the gills is present, often with the cartilage exposed. There is often secondary gill disease present, indicated by high numbers of bacteria or gill flukes. Lastly, the eyes are often sunken.

Treatment options at present are limited. Covering antibiotics and surfactants such as chloramine-T may be of benefit. Those fish that survive to go on and recover appear to be solidly immune to further infections. It may be that some of these become carriers of the virus, although experimentally recovered koi failed to pass on KHV to other, non-exposed koi.

A KHV outbreak in full swing is very difficult to confuse with any other infection. The combination of selective die-offs of koi with the characteristic gill damage makes it unlike any other disease. SVC can cause similar large die-offs, but the picture is different. Poisonings can do this too, but again the overall picture is different. It is only early on in the outbreak, where maybe one or two fish alone are ill, that KHV may be mistaken for another disease.

Prevention of KHV is difficult. It is not known at present how the virus can be transmitted, so it may be possible to transfer it on clothes, nets, plants, and so on. At the time of this writing, it is best to assume that this is a possibility. Some koi producers are attempting to "vaccinate" koi before selling them. This is done by exposing koi to the virus at 76°F for three to five days and then transferring them to water held at the non-permissive temperature of 86°F. These fish are resistant when challenged by infection due to high levels of virus-specific antibodies in their blood. They will be immune to further outbreaks, but some *may* act as carriers.

### Deep Angelfish Disease

This herpes viral disease appears to infect only the deep angelfish (*Pterophyllum altum*). Outbreaks are triggered by stress, and affected fish show loss of balance, spiraling behavior, and death. In an outbreak described, affected altum angels were kept with the common angelfish (*P. scalare*). It was not determined whether the herpes virus was specific for the altum angels or whether it was transmitted from the other angelfish species, all of which remained healthy throughout the outbreak.

### Ramirez Dwarf Cichlid Virus

This viral infection of the dwarf cichlid (*Mikrogeophagus ramirezi*) causes uncoordinated swimming and muscle spasms, leading to temporary flexion of the spine. Other signs include respiratory distress, loss of appetite, and eventual wasting. Hemorrhages in the skin and eye can occur.

### Corona-like Virus in Koi

This virus, which has been isolated in Japan, produces a condition in koi very similar to bacterial ulcer disease. The virus has not, as yet, been diagnosed elsewhere, but it may explain why some outbreaks fail to respond well to antibiotic medications.

# Bacterial Diseases

Bacterial diseases are common in aquarium and pond fish and can be a source of great frustration. Many of the bacteria associated with disease in fish are naturally present in the aquatic environment, and so their elimination from the fish's captive environment is virtually impossible. It also means that they are a constant threat to the fish that must rely upon a fully

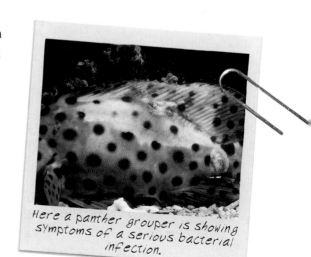

Here a panther grouper is showing symptoms of a serious bacterial infection.

functioning immune system to constantly fend off invasion by the pathogens.

## Common Bacterial Pathogens

Two recognized fish pathogens are *Aeromonas salmonicida achromogens* and those of the *Pseudomonas* complex, while opportunistic environmental infections include *Aeromonas hydrophila, Citrobacter,* and *Edwardsiella.* Occasionally, mixed infections of these bacteria may occur. It is thought that in some cases *A. s. achromogens* attaches and causes an initial lesion but is then swamped out by secondary invasion with other species.

Anything that stresses the fish or otherwise compromises its immune system may leave it open to infection. The usual suspects would include water quality, low or rapidly fluctuating temperatures, and overcrowding. Damage to the skin, which disrupts the protective mucous layer and breaches the outer layers of the skin, may allow these bacteria to attach and establish themselves on the exposed and damaged tissue. Such traumas may be physical: for instance, scale loss during the rough and tumble of spawning, or while scratching against objects. Scale loss may also be caused by large parasites. (A good example of this is the fish louse *Argulus.*) Poor nutrition also plays a part. High protein levels help to produce high antibody levels and essential fatty acids aid in antibody and white cell production, while vitamins A and C are also significant. Deficient diets mean an increased susceptibility to disease.

### What to Look For

Bacterial infections can potentially affect any ornamental fish. However, those that cause the most concern are koi and goldfish. It may be that these species have an increased susceptibility, or it could be that they are usually transported and kept in crowded conditions. In many establishments, goldfish seem to be treated as a commodity rather than as living organisms.

### Peracute

Usually this category is characterized by sudden, unexpected deaths with no obvious external signs. Microscopically there is often a massive overgrowth of one particular type of bacterium. The bacteria multiply so quickly that the fish is unable to mount any sort of an immune response. Death is usually due to toxins released by the infection. The infection could be confused with water-quality problems and poisoning.

*Common Bacterial Diseases Categories*

- Peracute (sudden)
- Acute (fast onset)
- Chronic (long term)

### Acute

These fish show classical signs of septicemia, with blood streaking and blotches (hemorrhages), especially on the skin and fins. Other symptoms are behavioral; the diseased fish lose their appetite, become sluggish, and clamp their fins. Infected individuals separate from the main group and will be found at the pond edges or aquarium corners. Again, many of these effects are a result of toxins released by the bacteria. Younger fish succumb first, and in a serious outbreak most of those affected may die. It is important to rule out parasitic infections as another possible cause of skin and fin hemorrhages. In a pond of koi and goldfish, another possibility would be SVC.

### Chronic

Ulcers in the body wall are probably the commonest presentation of a relatively long-standing or chronic bacterial infection. These can vary from being small, well-defined ulcers to extensive erosions of the body wall that can extend into the body cavity. Such ulcers are not just about the infection–they are a serious gap in the body's defenses that can allow other secondary invaders, such as fungi, to colonize the wounded tissue. Also, the fish suffer from the loss of body salts and an influx of water,

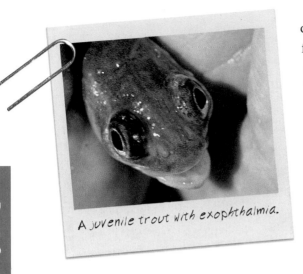

A juvenile trout with exophthalmia.

causing a marked dilution of body fluids. Such fish are unable to accurately control their fluid and salt balance, and in extreme cases or where there is also significant damage to the kidneys and/or gills, then a buildup of fluid inside the body cavity (ascites) can develop. In these cases the fish have a swollen abdomen, protruding eyes (exophthalmos), and scale protrusion. This latter sign gives the characteristic "pinecone" appearance of dropsy caused by the buildup of fluid in the scale pockets.

Occasionally, bacterial infections will be localized and present as a group of raised scales. Here infection has established in the scale pockets and has caused the individual scales to become more prominent. This can progress to true ulceration. Another presentation that can be seen is long-term muscle wastage, especially with the mycobacterium infections.

Gill necrosis due to bacterial gill disease in a koi.

Bacterial gill disease is another chronic manifestation involving bacteria. Here the bacteria are only part of the problem and gain a hold on the gills only after poor water quality has damaged these delicate tissues.

Clinical signs will be respiratory distress, heavy breathing, and hanging around areas with high oxygen levels. The gills may appear swollen and have discolored patches.

"When you are inspecting pond fish for ulceration, be sure to always net and bowl them to inspect their underbellies, as ulcers can be found lurking there and will be invisible from above."

In some cases it may be thought necessary for bacterial culture to be performed to determine the exact bacterium involved. A professional fish health expert using a sterile swab usually does this. In theory, the procedure should allow you to find out not only which specie or species of bacteria are causing the problem, but also to have it tested against appropriate antibiotics so that an appropriate treatment is started. The isolation of known secondary invaders such as *Aeromonas hydrophila* may not reveal the whole story, as it may have swamped out the true pathogen from the lesion.

Antibiotics are often the only truly effective treatments available, but they do have some practical drawbacks. Antibacterial proprietary medicines available from retail outlets are rarely effective against bacterial disease. Mild or early infections may occasionally respond, and the tea tree-based products are worth trying in these cases. For advanced bacterial infections, I find these products of little use, however.

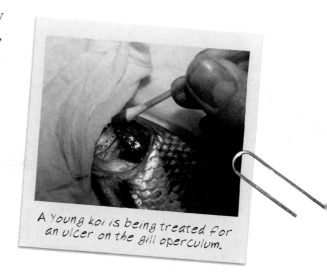

A young koi is being treated for an ulcer on the gill operculum.

Part 2

The presence of predisposing factors are also important–if the fish are stressed due to poor management, then no amount of medication will help them recover until their environment is corrected.

### Treatment

Individual fish may need injecting with an appropriate antibiotic. Groups or those that are still feeding may be given food impregnated or coated with an antibiotic. Before offering medicated food, starve the fish for 24 hours to make them hungry. If an antibiotic is available only as a tablet, crush the required amount until a powder is formed. Always wear gloves while doing this. Mix the antibiotic with a small amount of vegetable oil until it forms a thick paste. Mix this paste with an appropriate amount of pelleted food. Allow it to air-dry before feeding.

#### *Ulcers*

With the fish anesthetized, gently remove any devitalized tissue. Cotton wool pads are ideal for this. Gently apply a proprietary povidone-iodine compound, making sure to follow any dilution instructions. This iodine preparation is very good at antibacterial and antifungal properties. Then grout in a layer of medication used for treating mouth ulcers to act as an osmotic barrier while the ulcer heals.

*Injections are sometimes the only effective method for curing internal bacterial infections.*

Try to treat ulcers only once, as repeat treatments risk removing the delicate and easily damaged layers of cells that form as part of the healing process and so may slow down the rate of recovery. In all cases, especially if one is using proprietary off-the-shelf antibacterial preparations, speed of response is the most important thing. Your best chance of a successful outcome is to treat or seek assistance as soon as you realize there is a problem.

Diseases that may be mistaken for bacterial ulcer disease are fish tuberculosis (mycobacteriosis), sunburn, trauma, trichodiniasis, and hypersensitivity (allergic) reactions at attachment sites of

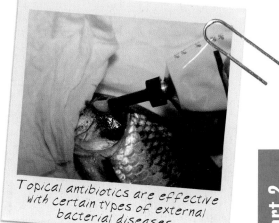

*Topical antibiotics are effective with certain types of external bacterial diseases.*

parasites such as *Argulus* and *Lernea* (anchor worm). In carp, SVC can mimic the hemorrhagic condition.

Avoid or correct any obvious predisposing factors. Water quality is of critical importance. Recently probiotic compounds have become available. These are preparations of beneficial bacteria that, once established in the pond or aquarium, reduce the numbers of pathogenic bacteria through a combination of competitive inhibition (these bacteria occupy the environmental space that the disease-causing microbes would normally inhabit) and the production of natural bacteriostats (bactocillins).

## Fish Tuberculosis (Mycobacterial Infection)

Fish tuberculosis is caused by a particular group of bacteria known as mycobacteria. The usual causes of mycobacteriosis are *Mycobacterium fortuitum*, *M. marinum*, and *M. chelonae*. These bacteria can be found as free-living environmental organisms, often in the mud and mulm that collects at the bottom of a body of water. A similar disease can be seen with another environmental bacterial contaminant called *Nocardia asteroides.* This is not a mycobacterium, but because the disease it causes is so similar to mycobacteriosis, it is usually considered alongside this group.

The usual means of infection is via the mouth, either by the fish grubbing around and feeding from the substrate, or by eating infected prey or cadavers. The mycobacteria then invade the gut wall, triggering the host's inflammatory response. Alternatively, cuts and abrasions can act as a doorway for infection. The best temperature for the growth of fish mycobacteria is around 74°F, with an average incubation period before the onset of clinical signs of around six weeks.

In the face of an infection, the immune system of the fish will attempt to contain and eliminate the mycobacteria by surrounding it with white blood cells bent on destruction of the invader. These aggregates of cells can be visible to the naked eye on postmortem fish and are called granulomas. They usually appear as gray-white nodules and can be found in a variety of organs. Unfortunately, this defense is often only partially successful. If one such granuloma erodes into a blood vessel, then mycobacteria can be carried to any structure or organ of the body.

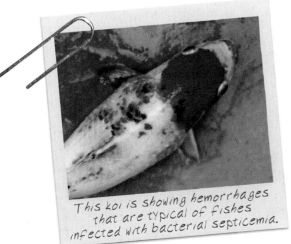

This koi is showing hemorrhages that are typical of fishes infected with bacterial septicemia.

The liver and kidneys are commonly infected because these are very active organs with a large blood supply. Granulomas develop in these organs. Infective material can then be passed out from the kidneys in the urine, while damage to the kidney itself may affect the ability of the fish to osmoregulate, so these fish develop a buildup of fluid in the body cavity (ascites or dropsy). If the liver is infected, mycobacteria can invade the gall bladder and bile ducts and can then be passed down into the gut along with bile to be eliminated in the feces.

Granulomas in the muscles of the body wall can erode outward to form skin ulcers. Infections in the brain may trigger abnormal behavior, while granulomas and fluid buildup behind the eyes can force them out of the sockets so that they noticeably protrude. Occasionally some mycobacteria will travel in the bloodstream to eventually lodge in one or more of the bones of the back. These vertebrae are eventually eroded away by the infection to such an extent that they collapse, causing obvious spinal deformities.

Serious damage to the guts and related organs such as the liver and pancreas will affect how the fish is able to digest and utilize its food, thereby causing a gradual wasting of bodily condition. The actual clinical signs that infected fish exhibit will reflect which organs are infected.

The presence of mycobacteria in the environment is an obvious predisposing factor, and they are probably very common. Infected fish will shed large numbers of infective bacteria into their surrounding water and onto the substrate, increasing the likelihood of any in-contact fish developing the disease. Stressors or concurrent disease processes that suppress the fishes' natural immune resistance will also increase the likelihood of infection. Mycobacteriosis is one of the main reasons why predatory fish should not be fed live feeder fish or "trash" fish as this. In fact, in addition to the scavenging of corpses, these are ideal ways of transmitting the infection. High stocking densities will increase the risk of infection. In platys (*Xiphophorus* spp.), the transfer of mycobacteria from a mother's infected ovaries into her unborn young has been demonstrated.

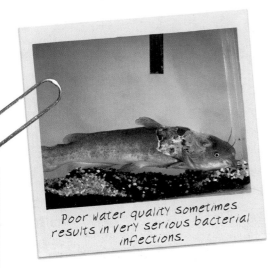

*Poor water quality sometimes results in very serious bacterial infections.*

## What to Look For

All species of fish are potentially susceptible, although this apparent susceptibility can vary. Cyprinids such as goldfish and tench (*Tinca tinca*), plus anabantids including the fighting fish (*Betta* spp.), paradise fish (*Macropodus* spp.), and gouramis (*Trichogaster* spp.) seem to be particularly susceptible. Aquatic reptiles, amphibians, and crustaceans can also harbor the disease.

Obvious signs of disease can be very variable depending upon where the infection has become established. Some fish will just waste away, while others will develop ascites.

Ulcers may form on the flanks and head. There may be an obvious exophthalmus (protrusion of the eye out of the socket) that can be one-sided, or both eyes may be affected. Sudden deformities of the spine may be seen. On postmortem fish, granulomas may be visible, often in several different organs. Always wear gloves if you are dealing with postmortem fish. Mycobacteriosis is potentially infectious to people and can enter through cuts in the skin!

## Treatment

Mycobacteriosis is highly resistant to the usual antimycobacterial medications. Certain antibiotics can be effective, but administering these treatments at an appropriate dose can be difficult and expensive. In addition, the aquarium or pond must be stripped out and thoroughly cleaned, which may include having to dispose of any gravel, plants, and decorations that cannot be reasonably cleaned and sterilized. The fact that it is potentially infectious to people does beg the question of whether we should treat it at all or whether humane euthanasia is the most appropriate action.

There is a wide range of clinical signs linked to this disease, and many parasitic, bacterial, and fungal diseases can mimic mycobacteriosis. In mollies (*Poecilia* spp.), *Flavobacteria* can cause multiple internal granulomas. *Aeromonas* or *Vibrio* bacterial infections can produce ulceration and signs of septicemia. *Ichthyophonus* is an internal fungal infection that can produce a progressive wasting condition, as can heavy internal parasite burdens such as with intestinal worm. Spinal deformities have been linked to a variety of conditions such as vitamin C deficiency in livebearers, such as swordtails (*Xiphophorus helleri*).

In orfe (*Leuciscus idus*), such deformities that occur following the use of certain medications are well documented. Electrocution, either from faulty aquarium electrics or from lightning strikes to ponds, appears to trigger a massive spasm of the strong back muscles, causing fractures of the vertebrae. To prevent this infection, quarantining of all new arrivals is a must. Prompt isolation of sick fish, along with the treatment of any problems, will help to eliminate other possibilities. Consider euthanasia of strongly suspect fish. In groups of susceptible fish, mycobacteria can thrive in aquaria, making its presence an important conservation issue with some captive breeding projects.

## Columnaris Disease (*Flexibacter columnaris*)

*Flexibacter columnaris* is a freshwater bacterium that belongs to a group of bacteria called cytophaga-like bacteria. Often shortened to CLBs, this group includes other pathogens, such as cytophaga and flavobacterium. Flexibacter columnaris is relatively long and slender; it is motile and tends to form large aggregates. Outbreaks tend to be temperature related and usually occur at more than 60°F. Fishes that appear healthy can carry this disease, and outbreaks will occur when conditions suit the infection. Ideal conditions include high temperatures and large amounts of organic waste. Flexibacter have been shown to grow on uneaten food.

Often the first sign of an infection is a largish white spot somewhere on the body. Soon it will develop a reddish outer tinge as the underlying skin becomes damaged and inflamed. This white spot is actually a mucoid exudate that contains tens of thousands of bacteria all massed together. Erosions appear, often with a reddened rim. Fins are frequently targeted, with the infection eroding the fins from the outside in toward the body. The gills are also affected, with extensive damage caused by the swarms of flexibacter. Other CLBs can secondarily invade at this point. The swimming pattern of the fish often changes at this point, and surface and mid-water swimmers begin a wobbling motion with exaggerated side-to-side movements of the tail. Eventually, the bacteria invade the bloodstream and there is a fatal spread to the internal organs.

Predisposing factors include water temperatures above 58°F and high levels of organic matter. Flexibacter do not appear to enjoy waters with a low pH and water hardness, although tolerances appear to vary among strains of bacteria.

## What to Look For

All species are potentially susceptible. The disease is well recognized in Japanese weatherfish (*Misgurnus augillicaudatus*), goldfish, carp, tilapia, and *Poecilia* livebearers, especially guppies and mollies. Large whitish patches on the body, gill covers, or fins may have a reddened rim around them. Discoloration or loss of body color is due to overgrowth of the infection. Respiratory distress, apparent by the rapid pumping of the gill covers and hanging at the surface, is a good indicator, too. Loaches may switch to alternative methods of breathing by swallowing air from the surface to be absorbed across the gut wall. Degenerate, ragged fins may be present, also known as classic "fin rot." Finally, there may be some blood streaking in the fins.

### *Mouth Rot or Mouth Fungus*

The bacteria, along with mucus and dead skin, will often hang from the mouth area. These strands may be seen moving (like hair) as the fish breathes. In guppies there is typically a simultaneous fin and tail "rot" along with white skin patches. Small, brightly colored tetras such as neons, cardinals, and glowlights may lose their color and develop whitish-gray patches. If you have access to a microscope, placing some of the whitish exudates onto a slide will reveal huge swarms of flexibacter. In some cases they can form a haystack-like appearance.

The most effective treatment is with antibiotics. Copper-based medications can work, as will surfactants such as benzalkonium chloride that act by helping to lift the bacteria off the gills and skin. However, flexibacter can be mistaken for many other bacterial infections. The whitish patches may be mimicked by a localized patch of excess mucus that is sometimes seen with some external parasitic problems. Fungal infections are another common misidentification. In small tetras, the loss of color and pale patches can lead to confusion with neon tetra disease or NTD (*Plistophora*).

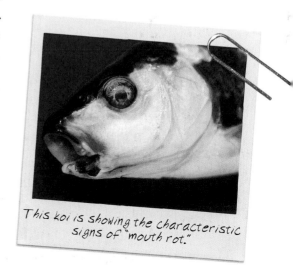

This koi is showing the characteristic signs of "mouth rot."

Part 2

Prevention can be difficult, as some fish are carriers yet show no signs of disease. Keeping the fish in optimal conditions and making sure that the amount of organic material is minimal should help to reduce the risk of infection.

### Epitheliocystis

Bacteria-like organisms that have yet to be properly classified cause epitheliocystis. They invade the mucous-secreting cells in the gills and skin of carp, triggering transparent or whitish cysts to form. If present in large numbers, these cysts can cause marked damage to the gills. Affected fish show respiratory distress because of the loss of functional gill tissue and a reactive excessive mucus production. Carp in particular show a proliferated reaction to infection–the surrounding tissues form a significant fleshy mass that looks like a small growth.

Infection is not common. When it does occur, it is usually associated with low temperatures and so probably needs an immunosuppressant to take root. However, epitheliocystis can easily be mistaken for the iridioviral infection *Lymphocystis. Lymphocystis* does not, however, infect carp and other cyprinids, though if you see a koi or goldfish with *Lymphocystis*, it most likely is epitheliocystis.

There is limited information available for the treatment of this disease. It may respond to certain antibiotics such as chloramphenicol, but the long-term use of this antibiotic may be immunosuppressive itself, so use caution when treating fishes with it.

### Piscirickettsia-like Organisms (PLOs)

Piscirickettsia-like organisms (PLOs) are another group of bacteria-like organisms. Little is known of them except that they have caused disease outbreaks in both cichlids and loricarid catfish. In farmed tilapia, outbreaks have caused death rates of up to 75% in some cases.

Infected fish become darkened in color, lose weight, and exhibit abnormal swimming behavior. In some cases there was thickening of the gill tissues (gill hyperplasia), and granulomas spread throughout the gills, spleen, and kidneys.

These PLOs have been experimentally transmitted from tilapia to another cichlid, *Parachromis managuensis*, which cohabited the same water. Fortunately, infections were unable to be triggered by injecting PLO-infected material into a variety of other cichlids, including red devils (*Amphilophus citrinellum*), freshwater angelfish (*Pterophyllum altum* and *P. scalare),* and *Cyphotilapia* spp., so it may prove to be a problem limited to only a few species. In blue-eyed panaques (*Panaque suttoni*) for example, the infection appeared to be triggered by the stress of transport during shipping.

An outbreak of PLOs is, at the time of this writing, an unlikely possibility. However, it should be considered if there are unexplained die-offs of tilapia, panaques, or other loricarids. This disease can be treated with a variety of antibiotics.

**Part 2**

# Fungal Infections

Fungal infections are a group of diseases that many hobbyists are familiar with, at least in theory. A wide variety of other diseases are mistaken for fungal infections, probably because many diseases can superficially mimic such an infection. In addition, fungi are common secondary invaders of wounds, and the blame is attributed to what is obviously seen. Treatment can be difficult–

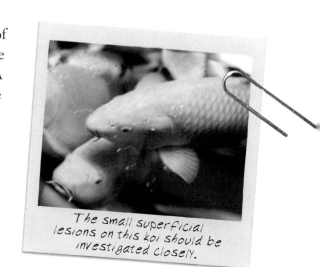

The small superficial lesions on this koi should be investigated closely.

fungi are not plants, and they possess many metabolic pathways that fish and other animals have. Targeting fungi can kill the fish as well as the fungus.

## *Saprolegnia* Fungal Disease

This is the most common fungal pathogen of freshwater ornamental fish. These fungi are usually saprophytes, which means that they normally feed and grow upon dead animal and plant material. If spores attach to a fish, normally substances in the mucous layer of the fish prevent their germination. However, if spores of this fungus find their way into a suitable place like a wound, they will germinate and send out branching stems called hyphae. These hyphae penetrate the skin and often spread into the deeper tissues. Eventually the fungus produces a set of hyphae to bear the fruiting bodies known as zoosporangia. It is from these that spores are released into the surrounding water. These raised hyphae give the classic "cotton-wool" appearance of a *Saprolegnia* fungal infection.

The fungus gets its sustenance from the fish, and in doing so causes extensive damage. Eventually the fish dies because the fungal infection damages the skin to the extent that the osmotic balance of the fish is disrupted, which means that the fish cannot maintain its body fluid and salt balance. On occasion the gills are targeted, often as a sequel to bacterial gill disease, where pathological changes to the gills favor lodging and establishment of fungal spores. Other fungal species do occur as opportunist pathogens and include the *Calytralegnia*, *Achlya*, *Aphanomyces*, *Dictyuchus*, *Leptolegnia*, *Pythiopsis*, and *Thraustotheca*.

### What to Look For

All freshwater species are potentially susceptible to a *Saprolegnia* fungal infection. The cotton wool-like patches are very characteristic and are often associated with areas of damage such as ulceration, and in extreme cases these fungal masses can completely envelop parts of the fish. In pond fish, fungal infections that have been present for some time may be green or brown due to secondary colonization by algae. Note that finding dead fish covered in fungal mats does not necessarily mean that the fish died from a fungal infection–spores are ever present, and *Saprolegnia* will rapidly establish itself on a cadaver. One particular manifestation of *Saprolegnia* is "staff's disease," where the fungal growths are present only in the nostrils. This is seen in common carp in Poland during the winter months in one to two-year-old carp.

For treatment, proprietary medications containing malachite green are strongly recommended. Remove any visible hyphae by swabbing the affected area with a 10% povidone-iodine solution once daily. Maintaining the fish in a salt solution will not only help to control the fungal infection, but it will also help with the osmotic imbalance resulting from the infection. Even salt solutions as low as 10 parts per thousand (mg/100mls) will inhibit *Saprolegnia* infections. Ideally, aim for 1 to 3g/l as a permanent solution until the problem has been resolved.

Colonies of the opportunist protozoan parasite *Epitsylis* can resemble patches of fungus. Microscopy will give a definite diagnosis. "mouth fungus" (along with fin rot) is often described as a fungal infection, especially in livebearers. This is not usually due to a fungal infection at all but a bacterial infection with the cytophaga-like bacteria such as *Flexibacter columnaris*. Excessive mucus production can look

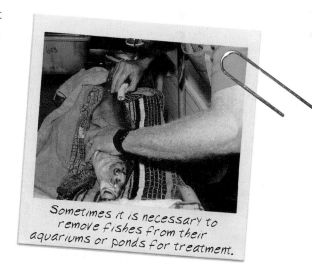

Sometimes it is necessary to remove fishes from their aquariums or ponds for treatment.

Part 2

remarkably like fungus, where the mucus hangs off the fish in strands. This is usually due to an ectoparasitic infestation or some other skin irritant. Fancy goldfish with well-developed hoods, such as lionheads and orandas, often have patches of whitish-colored mucus on their hoods. This is normal for these varieties.

## Ichthyophoniasis (*Ichthyophonus hoferi*)

Ichthyophoniasis is a fungal disease usually attributed to infections of *Ichthyophonus hoferi*. This disease can afflict both freshwater and saltwater fish and is considered to be the commonest reported fungal disease of marine fish. Fish become infected by accidentally eating resting infective spores. These can be present in the environment, but they can also be found in huge numbers in the bodies of dead infected fish. Most of these spores have many nuclei (**multinucleate**) and can divide into smaller endospores either by rupturing or by growing hyphae. These hyphae can then further subdivide to create more endospores. In some cases these endospores are able to move around like an amoeba.

After they have been consumed, partial digestion of the outer coats of the resting spore occurs, and they then penetrate the gut lining of host fish. The endospores are then disseminated throughout the body, possibly via the blood circulatory system, where they end up in those organs with a good blood supply, such as the liver, heart, and kidneys. The endospores develop further into larger resting spores that can be visible in the body as whitish nodules lying in the body cavity, or as yellowish or even black masses within affected organs. Microscopically there is a localized inflammatory response (**granuloma**) around these spores as the body attempts to wall off the spores. In some cases the

*"Fungal infections can usually be prevented by good husbandry; this is essential, as is rapid attention to any wounds."*

pigment melanin is deposited around such spores, giving rise to the black coloring described above.

The clinical signs that infected fish exhibit will vary depending upon how severe the infection is and which organs are affected. Sterility can result if the testes or ovaries are infected. One interesting effect of this disease is sex reversal seen in guppies; following infection of the ovaries in adult females, there appears to be an altered production of sex hormones, leading to a masculinization of these fish. The time course of the disease can be protracted, often lasting for many weeks to months before the fish succumbs. Dead or dying fish pose the greatest risk and these should be removed as soon as they are suspected to have the disease.

## What to Look For

Potentially, all species of fishes are susceptible. Freshwater fish, paradise fish, Siamese fighting fishes, tetras, barbs, goldfish, and guppies seem to be the ones most often infected. Wasting is common in spite of a generally good appetite. There may be a darkening of skin color, and obvious boil-like swellings can be seen on the skin. In extreme cases the skin may have a sandpaper effect as a result of a great number of granulomas present in the skin. Exophthalmia (protrusion of the eyes) may also be observed. Abnormal behavior and swimming patterns, such as corkscrew swimming, may be obvious if the central nervous system is invaded. These symptoms vary depending upon site of infection, but it often presents as a long-term wasting disease. Currently, there is no recognized treatment for this disease, as it appears to be resistant to the usual antifungal treatments.

Any wasting disease, such as fish tuberculosis (mycobacteriosis) or heavy intestinal parasitism, can mimic this disease. Skin ulceration can be caused by bacterial infections as well as by other fungal infections such as

Part 2

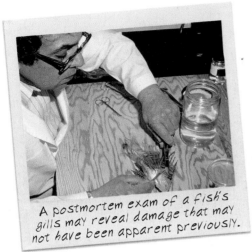

*A postmortem exam of a fish's gills may reveal damage that may not have been apparent previously.*

*Saprolegnia* and *Oomycetes*. The obvious internal cysts caused by *Ichthyophonus* sores could be mistaken for tumors or sporozoan cysts.

This is a disease best managed by control. Remove suspected fish and destroy them humanely. Scrupulous hygiene is important so that no spores survive in mulm on the aquarium bottom. Do not feed live food; always use gamma-irradiated (or otherwise sterilized) dead fish to carnivores.

## Gill Rot

Infection with the fungus *Branchiomycosis sanguinis* is occasionally encountered. Normally it occurs in natural ponds where there is access to mud and other organic materials for this fungus to survive off the fish. Infected fish will be seen to gasp at the surface and will appear weak and lethargic. Netting these fish and examining underneath the gill covers will often reveal raised areas of abnormal gill tissue. Sometimes there are greenish patches in the gills where algae are colonizing the fungus.

Gill rot is often fatal, but some fish recover and regenerate the damaged gill tissue. Predisposing factors include poor water quality, overcrowding, algal blooms, and temperatures of more than 68°F. At present there is no effective treatment, so it is best to concentrate on maintenance of optimum water quality, good food, and low stocking densities.

Part 2

# Protozoan Diseases

Protozoa are microscopic, single-celled animals. Protozoan diseases are common in fish, possibly because many of these organisms are naturally found to be present on the skin of fish in low numbers, and it is only when the immune system of the fish becomes compromised that numbers of parasites increase to problem levels.

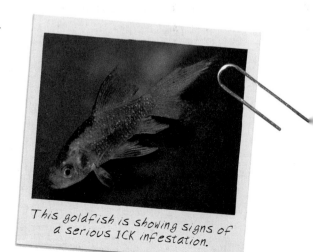

This goldfish is showing signs of a serious ICK infestation.

## External Protozoal Infestations

### White Spot or Ick (*Ichthyophthirius multifiliis*)

This parasite afflicts freshwater fish worldwide and is probably the most-often-diagnosed disease seen in aquarium fish. This is because it is very common and distinctive in appearance. The life cycle of *Ichthyophthirius* goes through several stages. The obvious white spots are cysts caused by individual parasites buried (and not just attached to) the skin and gills. Here they feed and enlarge. This parasitic stage is called a trophont. Eventually, the parasite ruptures out of this cyst and swims down to the bottom of the aquarium or pond. This stage is known as a tomont. Here it encysts again and begins to continually divide within the cyst, often forming up to 2,000 new free-swimming stages (theronts) of *Ichthyophthirius multifiliis*. When ready, the cyst opens and releases its contents into the surrounding water. These free-swimming stages must find a suitable host within 24 to 48 hours or else they will die.

The life cycle of *Ichthyophthirius multifiliis* is dependent upon temperature in two ways.

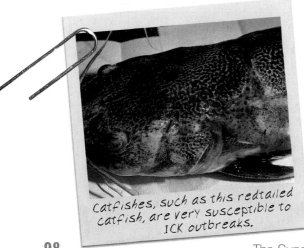

Catfishes, such as this redtailed catfish, are very susceptible to ICK outbreaks.

At higher temperatures the life cycle is completed quicker. At 82°F it takes around 6 days, 15 days at 60°F, and at 40°F it takes 35 to 40 days. This is important because in ponds the life cycle is still ongoing even at low temperatures; this can mean that parasite numbers gradually build up, giving the protozoan a numerical head start as waters warm up in the spring (at a time when the fish immune system is at its lowest).

More infective free-swimming theronts are produced at higher temperatures. Two and a half times as many are produced from an encysted trophont at 76° than at 70°F.

*Ichthyophthirius multifiliis* is a parasite that triggers a very good immune response in its host fish, so if the fish is not overwhelmed by a massive infestation, then not only will the fish recover well, but it will remain resistant to further outbreaks (providing it is otherwise healthy). The environmental encysted stage (*trophont*) is thought to be one of the means by which white spot is introduced into aquaria, attached to plants and gravel.

One of the most obvious factors linked with an outbreak of white spot is stress in one form or another. This may be a sudden cold snap (heater failure), transportation (in bag from shop to home), or any other event or disease that affects the fish's ability to raise an immune response. Because of the high degree of immunity in fish that have recovered from previous outbreaks, the spread of disease in an aquarium or pond may seem erratic. Some fish will suffer badly, often dying because they have had no previous exposure to the parasite. Others will show a few spots but will otherwise be unharmed, while others will show no signs of disease at all.

One classic scenario is that new fish are introduced into an aquarium, and a few days later there is an outbreak of white spot. The new fish die and some of the resident fish show some signs of illness. The aggrieved aquarist goes back to the shop claiming that he or she was sold sick fish. This may seem logical. After all, a fish, like a television set, should be fit for the purposes for which it is sold. However, in many cases the truth is that *Ichthyophthirius multifiliis* is already present in the home aquarium. The resident fish are immune and do not show signs. New fish with no immunity are introduced. The parasite finds susceptible hosts and rapidly multiplies its numbers to the stage where the new fish die and even the

**Part 2**

old fish show mild signs of disease. It is because of this that many aquatic outlets recommend routine treatment for white spot when introducing new fish.

### *Diagnostic Pointers*

All species of freshwater fish are potentially susceptible. The obvious sign is white spots (up to 1.0mm diameter) dotted around the surface of the fish. Usually distinct, in heavy infestations they may appear to merge together. Affected fish may show mild signs of irritation, or they may appear quite sick. Fins are clamped, and there may be a graying of the overall color due to excess mucus production in response to the irritation caused by the parasite. Ulceration and secondary bacterial infection may be obvious after the cysts have "hatched." In koi, one sees a "salt and pepper" dusting appearance with *Ichthyophthirius multifiliis* instead of the more common appearance.

In all fish, the gills are targeted, possibly because the free-swimming stages are drawn in and onto the gills during normal breathing. With some fish only the gills are affected, and one may only see fish with marked respiratory signs such as rapid, heavy breathing with wide opening of the operculum (gill cover). In many of these cases there may be no obvious signs of white spot on the skin. If you have access to a microscope, take a skin scrape and examine it. *Ichthyophthirius* is an obviously large protozoan with a horseshoe- shaped nucleus and a layer of cilia (tiny hairs) around it.

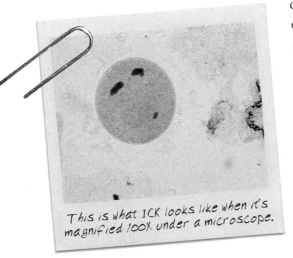

This is what ICK looks like when it's magnified 100X under a microscope.

This is a disease where many of the shop-bought remedies are effective in treating the condition. The active ingredient in these compounds is often methylene blue. However, methylene blue is effective only on the free-swimming stages, so treatment must be continued over an appropriate time course.

The trophont stage, buried in the skin, is relatively resistant to chemical attack. Repeat outbreaks are so common that it may be in many cases we are not eradicating the parasite completely, just stopping its rapid multiplication and allowing the fish's natural immunity to catch up and control the situation. Keeping the temperature high speeds up the life cycle, exposing the sensitive stages to medication sooner. It has been suggested that just raising the temperature and removing fish at a critical stage (before the free-swimming stages hatch to find a new host) can be done to eradicate the condition without using chemicals. I think this gives little credence to the versatility of this parasite and may unnecessarily stress fish with gills damaged during the infestation.

I have a feeling that it is highly likely that different encysted tomonts tick away on different internal clocks from each other, and they will release their infective free-swimming theronts at different times, irrespective of temperature. Some may even lie dormant for considerable periods of time. This, in my mind, is the only reasonable way to explain repeated recurrences of infestation in the same aquaria even after correct treatment. In the classic form of the disease, there is really nothing that looks quite like white spot.

Some sporozoan parasitic infections such as *Henneguya* do form "white spots," but these are larger and not quite so well defined as those seen with *Ichthyophthirius multifiliis.*

MERTHYR TYDFIL PUBLIC LIBRARIES

Part 2

Make sure to distinguish white spot from the small white nuptial tubercles on the operculae (gill covers) and the leading rays of the pectoral fins displayed by sexually active male goldfish.

Areas of ulceration may be mistaken as a bacterial infection only, with the possibility of an underlying white spot infection ignored. The respiratory signs seen with this parasite could be mimicked by poor water quality such as low oxygen levels. Other gill diseases, such as gill flukes and bacterial gill disease, should be considered.

Prevention is not easy, as the parasite is so common. Routine medication is one possibility, although I personally would not recommend this. Making use of a quarantine aquarium is an ideal way of preventing white spot from entering the main display aquaria or ponds. Newly attached trophonts will not be visible at first, but they should produce the characteristic white spots within a few days. Plants should be washed in a proprietary aquarium disinfectant before being introduced into an aquarium, while gravel/rocks and so on should be thoroughly dried and similarly disinfected before being transferred between aquaria.

Regularly rumors surface about the production of a white spot vaccine. Certainly this is a possibility, and experimentally it works. However, the low cost of individual fish, the relative ease with which white spot can be treated, and the sad overall pervading attitude that fish are a disposable commodity suggest that it would not be a good financial proposition.

### Tetrahymena

*Tetrahymena* causes so much trouble with livebearers that it is often referred to as the "guppy killer." It does, however, afflict other fish species, including tetras, scats (*Scatophagus* spp.), and cichlids. In large numbers, this ciliated parasite is intensely irritating, triggering mucus production and causing ulceration. These ulcers provide a portal of entry into the fishes' tissues, allowing the parasite to spread internally, especially to the eyes, muscles, and even into the brain and kidneys. In some cases the gills become severely damaged, leading to respiratory distress and death.

When *Tetrahymena* is buried deep in the tissues it is often resistant to treatment. *Tetrahymena* infestations also stress the fish and predispose them to secondary infections. *Tetrahymena* is often found in combination with other pathogens such as white spot (*Ichthyophthirius*) and *Flexibacter*.

### Diagnostic Pointers

This parasite particularly affects livebearers such as guppies and mollies but can infest other species, including cichlids. The fish will exhibit a clouded coloring due to increased mucus secretion and may even exhibit reddened patches, erosions, and even ulcers on the body surface and maybe even respiratory distress. Abnormal behavior such as odd swimming patterns (i.e. spiraling) can occur if the brain tissue becomes infected.

Treatment is usually straightforward, and commercially available medications should work. As an alternative, try chloramine-T at an average dose rate of 10mg/l, but remember to use less in soft water. Fortunately, concentrations even as low as 2mg/l may be of use in treating these infestations. *Tetrahymena* could be mistaken for other ectoparasitic infestations, including *Chilodonella* and *Trichodina*.

### Ichthyobodo necator (Costia necatrix)

*Ichthyobodo necator*, (or also known as *Costia*) is a very small protozoan parasite that is considered to be a normal skin inhabitant naturally found in very low numbers on the skin. It is quite mobile and is able to infest new hosts by attaching to the skin (including the fins) and the gills. It lives for only a few hours off the host. If the immune function of the fish is affected, then the numbers of *Ichthyobodo* can increase to levels where they become a problem. Initially affected fish appear depressed; their fins are clamped and they become anorectic. Ichthyobodo infestations appear to be very itchy, and infested fish will flick and scratch against objects and surfaces. Eventually, numbers can build to such an extent that the skin becomes damaged and allows secondary bacterial infections to occur, plus the gills are severely damaged. In some cases the gills only are affected. Such fish may be found dead with no outward signs of disease. Mass deaths can occur in an outbreak. *Ichthyobodo* is able to survive temperatures down to 38°F, and even at this low temperature, significant infestations have been described in hibernating carp.

### Diagnostic Pointers

All species of fish are potentially susceptible. Those species that are considered most prone to infection include goldfish, catfish, anabantids, swordtails (*Xiphophorus* spp.), killifish, and cichlids. Parasitized fish appear depressed and have their fins clamped shut. They may "wobble" as they swim, and the skin may appear dull in patches because the fish increases its mucous covering in response to the parasite. Progression to reddening or even ulceration of the skin can occur, due in part to the activities of the parasites, but also frequently the result of self-damage, as the fish scratch and flick against hard surfaces because of irritation. The infected fish will often exhibit respiratory distress, while some fish may have no obvious external signs.

Medicate with the standard proprietary antiprotozoan treatments. Raising the temperature to over 82°F will help to eradicate this parasite, but this will only help with species of fish able to cope with high temperatures, such as discus and fighting fish. Depopulating aquaria for 24 to 48 hours may be useful, as the parasite can only survive off the host for a few hours. Medicate the fish in a separate treatment aquarium. Outbreaks of *Ichthyobodo* can be confused with those of other ectoparasitic protozoa or flukes, all of which can all cause serious skin disease.

## Trichodina

*Trichodina* are protozoan parasites that are circular in shape with a layer of cilia rapidly beating around their circumference. Inside each parasite there is a concentric circle of "teeth" known as the denticulate ring. This is clearly visible, which in the living parasite can be seen to rotate. Viewed from the side, *Trichodina* has a dome-like shape. In reality there are at least three genera matching this description: *Trichodina, Trichodonella,* and *Triparciella* are seen in freshwater fish. These parasites reproduce by binary fission (dividing down the middle) and appear to be able to survive well off the host. No resistant spore is produced.

In low numbers these parasites are generally considered harmless, feeding upon suspended particles in the water or grazing across the surface of the skin, possibly consuming dead skin cells. In large numbers they are irritants and can cause serious damage to the skin. During outbreaks, *Trichodonella* and *Triparciella* often invade the gills, where they cause severe damage to the gill lining. In rare cases internal infestations have been described, with parasites being found in the kidneys, oviducts, and intestinal tracts. *Trichodina* is

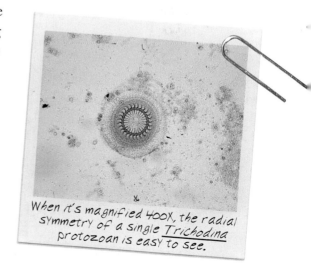

When it's magnified 400x, the radial symmetry of a single *Trichodina* protozoan is easy to see.

often found in the company of other ectoparasites such as *Gyrodactylus* (skin flukes) and other protozoa.

Trichodiniasis is more likely to occur with poor water conditions along with high levels of suspended faecal and mulm particles. High stocking densities increase the parasite's ability to move on to new hosts at a quicker rate. This parasite can be introduced into aquaria and ponds on plants and substrate materials such as gravel.

### Diagnostic Pointers

All fish appear to be susceptible. Experience suggests that it is a more common problem in koi and goldfish than with tropical aquarium fishes. This may reflect the way the former fishes are handled throughout the hobby. Infested fishes produce excessive mucus and so have a grayish cast. Skin erosions can form, which may lead to true ulceration.

The gills are usually badly affected also. In some cases, infestations may be limited to the gills alone. Affected fish will scratch against objects (flashing) and may show labored breathing or inflamed gills.

Treatment is fairly straightforward, as no resistant lifecycle stage is encountered. Begin by correcting any predisposing factors (i.e. poor water quality) and treat with any proprietary products containing formalin. Another option is to give the fish a salt bath at 10 to 15g/l for 20 minutes. This can be repeated daily if required, but it will only deal with parasites on the fish, not those in the aquarium or pond environment. As always, be cautious when using formalin with fish that show severe gill problems, as it can make the situation worse. There is much to be said for using an antibacterial product at the same time, as the lesions produced by the parasites commonly become secondarily infected.

Any disease or condition that triggers excessive mucus production can mimic *Trichodina* infestation. This would include other ectoparasitic diseases and poor water quality. Gill flukes (*Dactylogyrus*), low oxygen levels, bacterial gill disease, and so on can all cause respiratory distress that could be mistaken for this protozoal infestation of the gills.

Quarantining of new fish should help to prevent the introduction of *Trichodina*. Even transferring infested fish to a clean, good-quality environment can in some cases affect a cure. Pretreat all incoming plants with either a very dilute potassium permanganate solution or a proprietary aquatic disinfectant.

## Chilodonella

*Chilodonella* is a large protozoan parasite that has an almost oval, flattened appearance. It is very mobile, being well equipped with hair-like cilia that it beats to generate movement—a gliding, slow, circular movement.

*Chilodonella* is probably a natural part of the microscopic fauna that is present on the skin of many fish species. Normal parasite numbers are low, but if conditions favor the parasite, then buildup can be rapid. *Chilodonella* reproduces by division, and because these protozoans graze on the epithelial (lining) cells of the gills and skin, in large numbers they begin to cause damage. In the gills there is a reactive hyperplasia— a protective thickening of the delicate gill tissues that unfortunately causes a twofold problem.

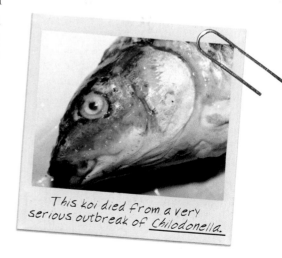

This koi died from a very serious outbreak of *Chilodonella*.

As the lamellae on the gills thicken, the spaces between them narrow. This reduces the amount of oxygen-carrying water that passes over them. These narrow spaces become gummed up with mucus and bacteria, which markedly reduces the total surface area for oxygen absorption and can allow secondary bacterial or fungal infections to establish in the gills.

The irritation of the skin results in an excessive mucus production as the fish attempts to shed the parasite by wrapping up their bodies in mucus. Infested fish often have clamped fins and appear depressed. Death usually follows due to excessive and irreparable damage to the gills.

The most significant predisposing factor is temperature–*Chilodonella* species prefer lower temperatures, and outbreaks are more likely to occur when fish are exposed to the low end of their temperature tolerance. In general, *Chilodonella* prefers temperatures of 68° to 72°F, but for some species (*Chilodonella cyprini* in particular), temperatures of 40° to 50°F seem to be close to their optimum. In pond fishes, these parasites can be a particular problem in the spring when the lower water temperatures give them a significant head start on the fish's immune system. Overcrowding can also be a factor in disease outbreaks and poor water quality both negatively affects the fish and while helping the parasite.

### Diagnostic Pointers

A wide variety of fish species are susceptible to *Chilodonella*. Groups that are particularly affected are the cyprinids, including goldfish and koi, but also barbs (*Puntius* and *Barbus* spp.), freshwater sharkminnows (*Labeo* spp.), and rasboras; cichlids, especially the Central and South American species, including the angelfish (*Pterophyllum* spp.), Ramirez's dwarf cichlid (*Mikrogeophagus ramirezi*), and the *Aequidens* group. Livebearers of the *Poecilia* (guppies and mollies) and *Xiphophorus* (swordtails and platys) genera are also occasionally affected. Mormyrids such as the elephant-nose

**Part 2**

fish (*Gnathonemus petersii*) can also be highly susceptible to infestation.

Typical signs of disease include respiratory distress and so-called "turbidity of the skin." Respiratory signs include increased breathing rate; the gill covers move faster and are extended much wider in order to maximize the flow of water over the compromised gills.

*Discus fishes are very susceptible to outbreaks of external protozoans.*

The fish may hang around at the surface or seek areas with relatively high oxygen layers such as filter outlets.

Formaldehyde (Formalin) is the medication of choice. In the first instance, use a proprietary ectoparasitic medication, the majority of which utilize formaldehyde in their makeup. Be careful with more "exotic" species such as the elephant nose and other morymids, as they may not respond too well to the formaldehyde. Make sure the water is well oxygenated, because formalin can have a direct effect on the gills–this is not a good thing when the gills of the fish are already seriously compromised.

Other treatments involve straight formaldehyde at 25ppm, followed

*"The skin turbidity is due to a dramatic increase in skin mucus production in response to the irritation caused by the parasites. When affected fish are removed from the water this mucus can form into gray gobbets of mucus."*

by a water change in four to eight hours or adding salt at 3g/l until symptoms stop. The use of surfactant compounds such as chloramine-T may be useful to help remove the thickened layers of mucus from the gill lamellae, but should be used with care. Saltwater baths should be considered for potentially sensitive fish. Antibacterial medication may also be necessary at the same time to prevent secondary infection of damaged areas of gill and skin.

Many ectoparasitic diseases such as *Trichodina* or flukes could mimic Chilodonellosis. Also, poor water quality can trigger the excessive mucus production so often seen with this disease. Quarantine will help to prevent the introduction of this parasite into your collection. If appropriate, then treatment with a formalin-based ectoparasiticide would be a good idea at this point. Also, maintaining optimum water quality– including temperature–is essential to reduce the risk of an outbreak.

### Velvet Disease (*Oodinium*)

*Oodinium* is a protozoan parasite, and just like green plants, this parasite is able to photosynthesize in the presence of light. The life cycle bears many similarities to that of white spot (*Ichthyophthirius multifiliis*). The infective stage (called a *dinospore*) swims until it meets a host fish, whereupon it attaches either to the delicate gill tissues or the skin. It sends out root-like projections deep into the skin, and there it stays, feeding and growing. This invasion triggers an inflammation with bleeding and thickening of

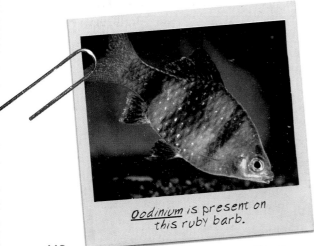

*Oodinium* is present on this ruby barb.

the skin at the affected areas. After three to seven days, the root-like processes are withdrawn and the parasite forms a protective cyst around itself and then falls off the host to settle in the substrate. Next it divides many times inside the cyst until over 200 spores are eventually produced. Each will eventually become a motile **dinospore**. These hatch out

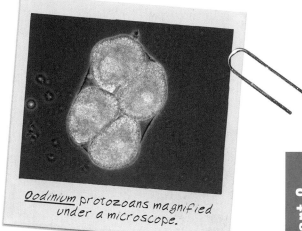

*Oodinium* protozoans magnified under a microscope.

and seek new fish hosts, although they can only last up to 12 to 14 hours without finding a host before dying. The whole life cycle can take up to ten days, but it is usually much shorter at higher temperatures. Serious infestations can rapidly build up within a few days, causing heavy losses. If you suspect this disease, do not hang back with treatment.

High stocking densities and high temperatures can lead to a rapid rise in parasite numbers. High light intensity may also favor this parasite, as it is able to survive off the fish by utilizing its chloroplasts.

### Diagnostic Pointers

All species can become infected but freshwater anabantids, such as the round-tailed paradise fish (*Macropodus ocellatus*), goldfish, White Cloud Mountain minnows (*Tanichthys albonubes*) and some killifish seem to be especially susceptible. The chloroplasts impart a brownish-greenish coloration to the parasite that can be seen with the naked eye. In large numbers, this coloring imparts an impression of a velvety texture, hence the common name of velvet disease.

Part 2

Infested fish will often show very labored breathing from gill damage. There is often an excessive mucus production of the skin accompanied by scratching and flicking. Reddened areas of hemorrhage and ulceration occur where the skin has been damaged by the encysted stages leaving the fish. *Oodinium* has also been recorded as a serious parasite of aquatic amphibians, infecting such animals as newts and the tadpoles of various frog species.

Part 2

Treatments that are formaldehyde or copper-based are usually effective, but recurrent outbreaks can be common because the encysted stage is relatively resistant to chemical attack. Also, the parasite can colonize the intestines of fish, where it can be further protected from medications. In these cases, treatment with the antibiotic metronidazole can be used at a dose rate of 50mg/l daily for ten days, changing the water daily. Although metronidazole is considered an antibiotic, it is often an effective antiparasitic and antiflagellate medication as well. In severe outbreaks, antibiotic cover ointments should be considered because secondary infections are common in those areas where the skin has been damaged.

It may be possible to eliminate the parasite from an aquarium by removing all of the fish, reducing or cutting out the light levels and raising the temperature to 82° to 86°F for three weeks. This will speed up the protozoa's life cycle in such a way that all the encysted stages will release their motile infective dinospores only for them to die because there are no hosts available.

The velvety appearance of *Oodinium* is characteristic, but other external parasites could mimic the excessive mucus production, irritation, and respiratory signs. Bacterial infections may cause similar damage to the skin. Quarantining all newly acquired fish for a period up to four weeks can prevent *Oodinium*.

# Internal Protozoal Infestations
## *Spironucleus vortens*

*Spironucleus vortens* is the cause of a range of diseases, including hole-in-the-head (HITH) or head-and-lateral-line (HLL) disease of discus. *Spironucleus* generally lives in the gut, and if something affects the fish's immune system (such as stress, poor diet, overcrowding etc.), then the parasites' numbers will build up. It appears to be able to cross the gut wall and spread via the bloodstream to anywhere in the body, including the spleen and ovaries. The liver has a huge blood supply and so it is frequently targeted in these cases as well. Damage to the gut wall affects the ability of the fish to digest and absorb its food. Infected fish lose weight and pass white, jelly-like feces.

HITH and HLL are possibly caused by the parasites inadvertently blocking the blood vessels to the lateral line causing tissue death and ulceration of those areas supplied by the affected blood vessels. In some cases *Spironucleus* can be found in these head lesions.

### *Diagnostic Pointers*

All species of cichlids may be potentially susceptible, but the most susceptible species appear to be discus (*Symphysodon* spp.) and angelfish (*Pterophyllum* spp.). Other cichlids that can be affected include Oscars (*Astronotus* spp.) and flower horn cichlids. Affected fish will often darken in color and go off their food. They may appear wasted, and discus may develop a pinched-gut appearance. Feces appear white and jelly-like.

Erosive holes begin to appear on the head, usually associated with the lateral line. The small pores that form the lateral line enlarge and may fuse. Often there is a whitish, stringy discharge from the pores. In some cases large areas of skin may be affected. Treatment of choice is with metronidazole. Dimetridazole has been used in the past, but there appear to be problems with sterility in fish once this medication has been used.

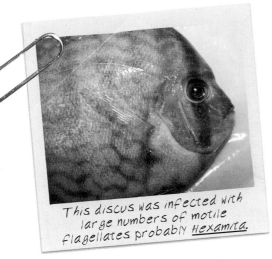

This discus was infected with large numbers of motile flagellates probably Hexamita.

## Hexamita

*Hexamita* is a protozoan that is often confused with *Spironucleus*, and indeed it is very difficult to tell the difference between the two under a microscope. As a result, there is much confusion between the two in the literature. I think there is, however, enough information to distinguish the two disease entities. *Hexamita* is known to cause particular problems in cichlids and anabantids.

*Hexamita* is an inhabitant of the gut, and its numbers can increase if the fish's immune system is suppressed. Infected fish become anorexic, lethargic, and lose weight. Other fish may develop a dropsy-like condition with swelling of the body cavity. *Hexamita* can spread via the bloodstream, causing a disseminated hexamitiasis.

### Diagnostic Pointers

Many fish species can be affected, but with ornamental fish it is usually cichlids and anabantids that suffer the majority of cases. Cichlids, discus, angelfish, and Oscars (*Astronotus* spp.) are particularly affected. In the Siamese fighting fish (*Betta splendens*), *Hexamita* can cause dropsy-like signs due to multi-organ damage. The liver and kidneys are especially affected. In kissing gouramis (*Helostoma temmincki*), *Hexamita* has been linked to swimming abnormalities, emaciation, white stringy feces, and secondary bacterial infections of the skin.

Fish lose their appetite and become thin and lethargic. Severely affected angelfish will show a distended abdomen and may lie flat at the water

Part 2

surface. Less severely affected adult cichlids may have reduced fertility, egg hatchability, and increased loss of fry.

Treatment is most effective with metronidazole at 50mg/l as a bath for up to 24 hours daily for ten days. As an alternative for fish that are not feeding, metronidazole can be administered in a bath at a concentration of 5mg/l every other day for a total of three treatments.

In certain systems, such as retail and wholesale outlets, *Hexamita* may become established to the extent that any new fish placed into the system may become challenged and may come down with disease. Such cases are particularly difficult to manage, as there is often a high turnover of stock that gives a constant supply of naive and stressed fish for the parasite to colonize. Prevention may be obtained by quarantining all new stock, possibly with routine medication during this period.

## Cryptobia

*Cryptobia iubilans* is a protozoan parasite that is thought by many to be the main culprit behind "Malawi bloat," a poorly understood condition not only of Rift Lake cichlids (Malawi, Tanganyika, and Victoria) but also transmissible to Central and South American cichlids. *Cryptobia iubilans* makes its home in the gut. Interestingly, this parasite has been found present in the stomach and gut of freshly caught wild *Metriaclima zebra*.

The main damage caused by this parasite is that it triggers inflammatory reactions (granulomas) in the lining of the stomach; in some cases it can spread to involve the liver, kidneys, brain, and other organs. If the liver and kidneys become involved, then a buildup of fluid in the body cavity can occur causing an apparent "bloat." In many cases I have seen there has been no bloat–often these fish are wasting away!

The actual triggers for an outbreak are not entirely known, but it is believed that several factors can trigger disease. These include poor water quality, stress, and handling. Diet almost certainly plays a role in herbivorous cichlids. Failure to provide sufficient vegetable material in the diet of mainly herbivorous cichlids may produce an altered gut environment that allows the *Cryptobia* to cause problems.

### Diagnostic Pointers

All cichlid species are potentially susceptible. It is a particular cause of mortalities in the Rift Lake cichlids but has been transferred to Central American cichlids, including the firemouth (*Thorichthys meeki*) and Nicaragua cichlid (*Hypsophrys nicaraguensis*), as well as South American species such as severums *(Heros* spp.)*.

The main sign of infection with *Cryptobia* is a progressive loss of appetite. Infected fish separate themselves from the main group. These fish eventually become so anemic that they hang at the surface. There is a markedly high respiratory rate followed by death within 24 hours of this stage. In some collections, virtually all the cichlids can be infected, and the disease will show itself as a low-grade loss of fish over a period of time.

There is no effective treatment, although some antibiotics such as metronidazole appear to be useful in controlling outbreaks. The postmortem picture of multiple granulomas is impossible to distinguish from fish tuberculosis without specialist laboratory techniques.

Quarantine all new cichlids for around four weeks to allow them to adjust to their new diet and conditions before introducing them into an established collection. Try to provide a good substitute diet, especially for herbivorous fish such as the mbuna.

## Sporozoan Parasites

This group of parasites contains groups of internal protozoa that are, to be honest, poorly understood. In some cases we do not know how fish become infected, what triggers an infection, or even how much damage they actually do. The one that most is known about is *Plistophora hyphessobryconis*, also known as neon tetra disease (NTD).

### Neon Tetra Disease

The cause of neon tetra disease (NTD) is the sporozoan parasite *Plistophora hyphessobryconis*. This parasite appears as accumulations of spores in the muscle tissue causing damage. Muscle fibers become replaced by accumulations of spores. These accumulations become visible to the naked eye as whitish patches that also cause a loss of the overlying skin color. *Plistophora* is relatively common in the neon tetra (*Paracheirodon innesi*), where it causes a loss of the blue body color that makes the reflective flash along the side and tail, replacing it with whitened, infected tissue. These patches of abnormal tissue can affect the swimming ability of the fish. In fish such as angelfish, the parasite triggers an immune response involving black pigment-bearing cells called melanophores. It is unknown how this parasite spreads, although it could be through eating contaminated or infected live and frozen food or by scavenging infected dead fish.

### *Diagnostic Pointers*

*Plistophora* it can affect tetras, barbs, rasboras, and angelfish. I have seen similar problems in guppies and killifish (*Aphyosemion australe*). In neon tetras and related fish, there is a loss of normal body color. White patches appear in the tissue of the affected areas. Normal swimming patterns may be lost. Fish close to death often become bloated, although this is likely due to secondary infections. It is common for most of a group of neon tetras and related fish to become sequentially infected and die.

In angelfish the areas of muscle damage and loss produce an uneven skin surface. In white angelfish there is often an obvious accumulation of melanophores at these areas producing a condition sometimes known as "black holes." This disease is not commonly fatal in angelfish although these fish become deformed.

There is no appropriate treatment. In the face of an outbreak, it is best to remove dead fish and euthanize obviously infected fish as soon as they are spotted to help prevent the disease from spreading. The most likely diseases to be confused with *Plistophora* are mycobacteriosis and columnaris (*Flexibacter*) infections. Mycobacterial granulomas in the muscle can resemble *Plistophora* spores, while *Flexibacter* causes a whitish skin discoloration reminiscent of *Plistophora* at first glance.

## Other Sporozoan Diseases

A number of other sporozoan parasitic organisms have been described. *Shaerospora renicola*, for example, is a parasite that causes swim bladder inflammation in carp fry. Affected fish lose their balance and can stop feeding. Those that survive to the following year are susceptible to bacterial infections of the swim bladder, as well as anemia and kidney swelling.

*Myxosoma dujardini* and *M. encephalina* are also found in carp. *M. dujardini* causes yellow-white cysts in the gills, leading to breathing difficulties and death, while *M. encephalina* infects the blood vessels of the brain, triggering behavioral and swimming problems such as circling and spinning.

*Henneguya koi* attacks koi and manifests itself as small, smooth, rounded "cysts" or nodules in a variety of organs, especially the gills and skin. This is an intracellular parasite that forms large pseudocysts (the nodules) from which large numbers of spores are eventually released. This happens at

**Part 2**

the death of the fish, although skin nodules may rupture. It is best to remove affected individuals, as they may pose a risk of infection.

*Eimeria carpelli* and *E. subepithelialis* both cause significant disease in young carp. Losses are seen in the early spring (before the carp start to feed), with those surviving showing marked weight losses. The most severe disease is caused by *E. carpelli.* It damages the lining of the bowel, causing severe enteritis with reddened gut lining.

In addition, *Eimeria macropoda* and another *Eimeria* sp. have been found in the intestines of the round-tailed paradise fish (*M. ocellatus*) and three-spot gouramis (*T. trichopterus*), respectively.

A cryptosporidium-like parasite (*Piscicryptosporidium reichenbachklinkei*) has been described in the pearl gouramis (*Trichogaster leeri*), while the related *P. cichlidaris* is known to infect cichlids (*Oreochromis* spp.). These are of uncertain significance, but it appears that these parasites imbed themselves in the lining of the stomach, giving them the potential to do much damage.

### *Hofferellus* sp.
#### (also known as *Mitaspora*)

*Hofferellus cyprini* causes kidney disease in carp and koi. Badly infected fish lose weight and die after around 7 to 14 days. Conversely, *H. carassii* is found in the kidneys of goldfish and triggers a massive growth of the kidneys, turning them into huge,

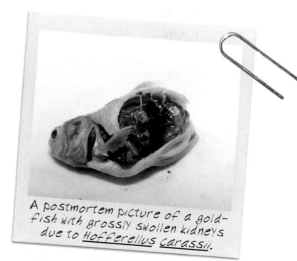

A postmortem picture of a goldfish with grossly swollen kidneys due to *Hofferellus carassii.*

Part 2

fluid-filled structures. In both cases, infected tubificid worms transmit the *Hoferellus* species.

For many of these diseases there are no effective treatments. *Eimeria* may respond to sulphonamide antibiotics or to anticoccidial drugs such as amprolium as a continuous bath at 10mg/l for seven to ten days.

# Worms and Flukes

A wide variety of parasitic worms species infect fish. It's a good life—the worms are protected and nourished by their host and in some cases appear to cause no problems to their host fish. There are cases, however, when worms can cause harm to their host.

Food material is usually broken down in the stomach and guts of the host fish into simpler, easily

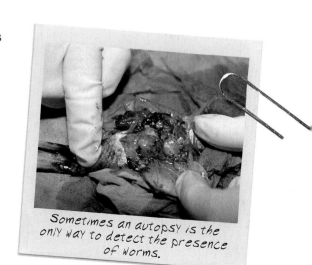

Sometimes an autopsy is the only way to detect the presence of worms.

absorbed substances such as sugars and amino acids. These are also what the parasites need in order to fuel their own metabolism and reproduction, and so there is direct competition between the host and the parasite. If the parasite is present in large numbers, then the fish may not be able to absorb enough of its own food across the gut wall before its parasites have taken it, causing a severe loss of body condition in the host despite an often increased appetite.

The presence of parasites in the gut may trigger an inflammatory reaction in the gut wall. This may trigger a thickening of the gut wall that in turn affects the ability of the host to absorb food across it at that point. More serious damage can also be done that can lead to blood loss (with an accompanying loss of important blood proteins and salts). Thorny headed worms especially may cause extensive damage with the array of hooks attached to their heads, causing hemorrhagic enteritis that can be a very debilitating illness. The damaged areas of the bowel are also unable to absorb food across them, thus reducing the total gut surface area available for food absorption.

Large tapeworms can be many centimeters long and are often folded back upon themselves in the fish's gut. Roundworms can form large aggregations in the gut. Both of these situations can lead to a partial or complete blockage of the gut.

There may be other consequences of a gut parasite infestation. Some species of roundworms will occasionally penetrate through the gut wall and carry infection from gut bacteria with them. In other groups of animals, allergies to gut parasites are suspected to be significant, and something similar may prove to be the case with ornamental fish.

# Roundworms (Nematodes)
## Capillaria

*Capillaria* are roundworms that have been recognized for a number of years to be a serious problem in discus, although they can occur in other species. The general opinion is that discus are particularly sensitive to infestations with this worm, a parasite from which they seem to be free in the wild. The numbers present in the gut can reach relatively large proportions, causing an obstruction and outcompeting the host discus for its food. Infested fish lose weight, although their guts may be so impacted with worms that the abdomen appears bloated.

Adult female *Capillaria* lay eggs that are passed out in the feces of the fish. Other fish become infected by accidentally eating these eggs. Intermediate hosts such as invertebrates may be important for this transfer. The worms compete with the host fish for nutrition and can cause gut obstructions. In addition, it is thought that these worms damage the lining of the gut, thereby allowing protozoa such as *Spironucleus* and *Hexamita* to invade the rest of the body.

### Diagnostic Pointers

Many fish may carry these worms, but discus (*Symphysodon* spp.) appear to be particularly prone to infestation. Emaciation is one of the primary indicators of the presence of *Capillaria*. This is best identified by the loss of muscle over the back, and the backbones can become very prominent. The abdomen may bulge because of the huge worm burden, and white, stringy feces may be passed. Typical *Capillaria* eggs (almost urn-shaped) will be seen if fecal samples are placed under a light microscope. Treatment is with routine worming as described for *Camallanus*.

## Camallanus

*Camallanus* are small, red-colored, parasitic thread-like roundworms (or nematodes). The adult worms are found in the intestine, colon, and

Part 2

rectum and can reach up to 1.0cm long. The female worm, which can often be seen protruding from the anus of infested fish, lays its eggs into the general aquarium environment. An embryo develops inside each of these eggs, and there it rests until the egg is eaten accidentally either by another fish or by a crustacean. The *Camallanus* worm now has two means of completing its life cycle.

In the first case, once the egg is eaten, the shell is digested and the now larval worm is released. It grows by molting several times before becoming a sexually mature adult. This is known as a *direct* life cycle.

In the second case, the egg hatches after being eaten by a crustacean (referred to as an intermediate host). This is often a copepod. The larval worm will then undergo several changes before being able to infect a fish (the final host), which it does when the parasitized crustacean is eaten. This is known as an *indirect* life cycle. *Camallanus* is often introduced into a collection following the feeding of infested live foods such as copepods, or by mixing with infested fish.

### *Diagnostic Pointers*

A wide range of species can be infested, but the commonest hosts are livebearers such as guppies, mollies, and swordtails. Killifish seem to be particularly affected in the presence of a *Camallanus* outbreak, possibly because of their small size or because they are more likely to eat copepods. A classic sign is a cluster of worms protruding from the anus of an infested fish. In smaller fish there may appear to be extensive damage and erosion around the vent area. Weight loss or a failure to thrive may be seen. There is an increased susceptibility to secondary infections, including tail and fin rot. The worms cause damage and ulceration of the lining of the gut, causing enteritis. This is shown as the passing of stringy or slimy feces.

Treatment is with various antihelminthic drugs such as Levamisole at 10mg/l as a single dose added to the water. This is particularly good for killing larval worms. Suspend carbon filtration and use piperazine at 2.5mg/g of feed, added to the food. This may only kill adult worms. Fenabendazole at 50mg/kg bodyweight added to feed or administered by stomach tube if the fish is large enough should also be effective. Fish are quick to refuse medicated food, so it is best to withhold food from them for 24 to 48 hours prior to offering such feed.

None of these medications are licensed for use in fish, and with the potential for their use in hundreds of different species of ornamental fish, their safety cannot be guaranteed in all species at all times. The obvious sign of a cluster of worms at the anus is very characteristic of *Camallanus* infestation, but other intestinal worms can cause weight loss, ill thrift, and enteritis. These would include *Capillaria* (another nematode worm) and tapeworms. Intestinal protozoan parasites can occasionally be encountered; the coccidian *Eimeria carpelli*, for instance, can cause severe enteritis in young carp. Deep-seated bacterial infections such as mycobacteria (fish tuberculosis), or fungal infections like *Ichthyophonus* could also cause a marked loss of condition.

## Thorny Headed Worms

Thorny headed worms (Acanthocephalans) are occasionally encountered, especially in Rift Lake cichlids and Australian native fishes. They each have a series of spines on their heads that help them to attach to the gut wall, but they can also easily damage the lining of the bowel. These worms have an indirect life cycle but it is usually, not always, in a fish in which the adult stage is

"Always quarantine and scrutinize all new fish for the characteristic red worms visible from the anus, and do not feed live copepods from unknown sources to fish."

**Part 2**

found. The intermediate stages are commonly found in invertebrates but can also be found in "prey" species of fish. Treat as for *Camallanus*.

## Flatworms (Cestodes)

Cestodes contain the groups of flatworms known as tapeworms and flukes. Tapeworms are often long, and their body consists of a series of segments, numbering from only three or four in the small species to hundreds in the larger. Flukes, also known as trematodes, tend to be relatively small and are not segmented. Flukes are divided into two groups.

The first group includes those that have a straightforward life cycle with only one host involved. These are known as monogenetic trematodes. The second group includes those with a complex life cycle involving different stages occurring in different species of animal. These are known as digenetic trematodes.

## Tapeworms

Tapeworms are flat worms that are usually attached by their head to the lining of the bowel. Some are relatively small, such as *Khawia* found in carp, while others can be very long, often longer than the whole length of the intestine! An example of this would be *Bothriocephalus*, another tapeworm of carp.

All tapeworms have an indirect life cycle, whereby eggs produced by the adult worm in the gut are passed out in the host's droppings, where they are taken in by one or more intermediate hosts. It is only after the main (primary) host fish has eaten the intermediate host that the adult worm finally develops and the life cycle is completed. This indirect life cycle means that tapeworms parasitize fish in two different ways. If the fish is the primary host, then these worms live as adults in the intestine and can cause similar problems to those seen with the roundworms. In *Khawia*, tubificid worms are intermediate hosts, while in *Bothriocephalus*, copepods play this role. However, for many tapeworm species the fish is an intermediate host, with a fish-eating bird often playing the role of a primary host. In these cases the tapeworms are present as encysted, intermediate stages in the muscle or body cavity of the fish. These encysted stages in their most benign form just sit and bide their time. In some cases the intermediate stages can enter the brain first, altering their host's behavior to make them more noticeable to predators.

The complex life cycle of tapeworms means that they rarely cause problems in aquaria where the life cycle is unlikely to be completed. Most tapeworm problems are therefore encountered in wild-caught or pond-reared fish, especially livebearers such as guppies. An effective treatment is praziquantel as a three-hour bath at 10mg/l, or 400mg/100g food once daily for seven days.

## Skin Flukes (*Gyrodactylus* species)

Skin flukes are flat worms of the genus *Gyrodactylus*. They are monogenic worms, which means that they have a direct life cycle so that an intermediate host is not needed for completion of the life cycle to adulthood. Generally they reach up to 0.8mm in body length, but occasionally one may see some very large (several millimeters long), highly pigmented ones on African fishes such as reed fish (*Erpetoichthys calabaricus*) and fahaka puffers (*Tetraodon fahaka*).

Gyrodactylids have at one end their characteristic large hooks that under the microscope are easily recognizable by the rough H-shape that the hooks form. *Gyrodactylus* are livebearers, and often the next generation of skin fluke can be seen inside the adult fluke. This mode of reproduction also means that numbers can build up rapidly if conditions suit them.

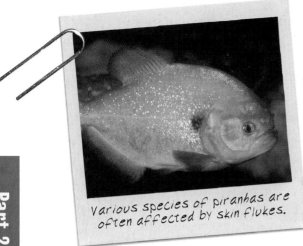

Various species of piranhas are often affected by skin flukes.

Part 2

They live on the skin of fish and graze upon skin cells and blood. They can cause direct damage to the skin of fish and allow secondary bacterial infections to enter. (The common fish bacterial pathogen *Aeromonas hydrophilai* has been isolated from gyrodactylids.) Skin flukes also cause problems indirectly by irritating the fish, causing it to scratch and scrape with the loss of the protective mucous layer, as well as the underlying skin layers. In heavy infestations, skin flukes can invade the gills.

Skin flukes are usually transmitted by direct contact between fish, but this is not essential. Contact with the bottom and sides of aquaria and ponds also contribute to rapid spread.

High stocking densities allow rapid spread of the infestation. Poor water quality and other stressors and illnesses lower the fishes' immunity, allowing infestations to establish.

### Diagnostic Pointers

As members of this genus are found in both freshwater and marine environments, all fish species are potentially susceptible. Irritation (the fish may be flashing) and reddened areas or a dullness of the skin associated with excess mucus production or even ulceration of the skin may occur. In some instances, fins may look ragged due to alternating areas of loss of tissue and localized reactive thickening of the skin.

These flukes are relatively large and can be seen easily on low power light microscopy of a skin scrape. Often they can be seen stretching and trying to move about. Look for the hooks–following treatment, these may be all that are visible. The hooks and lack of black "eye-spots" help to distinguish skin flukes from gill flukes.

### Treatment

Formalin-based medication using a proprietary treatment from your local aquatics outlet is recommended. Because they are livebearers, there is no resistant egg stage, which means that one treatment can potentially eliminate an infestation.

Saltwater baths conducted for five minutes daily over a period of five days may be beneficial. Praziquantel can be used for discus and smaller species of tropical fishes at a suggested dosage method with praziquantel is a one to two hour bath at 15 to 20mg/l. With larger fish such as koi, infeed medication at a rate of 400mg/100g food daily for seven days would be more appropriate. While generally effective, it has not been so successful with the larger flukes mentioned above. Other drugs that have proven to be useful include mebendazole and levamisole.

Organophosphates can also be used, but these are very tightly controlled in countries such as the United Kingdom. These must be used at the correct dose rates, as resistance to organophosphates has been recorded in some populations.

Skin fluke infestations can be confused with disease caused by other external parasites including protozoa and gill flukes (*Dactylogyrus* sp.). Water-quality problems may trigger an excessive mucus production that mimics an ectoparasitic problem. Hemorrhagic skins resulting from

MERTHYR TYDFIL PUBLIC LIBRARIES

bacterial infections may resemble an infestation. Small numbers are usually well tolerated by most fishes. Routine treatment during a quarantine period may be useful.

### Gill Flukes (*Dactylogyrus* species)

Gill flukes are generally microscopic, although some are just large enough to be seen by the naked eye. Along with their cousin, the skin fluke *Gyrodactylus* sp., they are grouped in the Class Monogenea, a subdivision of the flatworms.

Both the gill flukes and skin flukes are hermaphrodite (they contain both male and female sexual organs), but *Dactylogyrus* differs from *Gyrodactylus* in that they produce eggs, which are mostly shed into the environment. Like skin flukes, gill flukes have a direct life cycle. The temperature of the water governs reproduction of gill flukes, so that at 35° to 40°F, the life cycle is five to six months, while it is reduced to only a few days at 72° to 78°F. Adult flukes feed upon the cells of the gill tissue, blood, and the mucus produced in response to damage and irritation by the parasites.

This lionfish died of anoxia due to an infestation of gill flukes.

Higher temperatures speed up the reproductive rate of this parasite, so with temperate pond fish, gill fluke problems often occur in the warmer months. High stocking densities increase the chance of the free-swimming larval stage finding a host, providing an increased "hit rate."

### Diagnostic Pointers

All species of fish are potentially affected, although the actual species of parasite (and the amount of damage it causes) can vary. In freshwater fish it is usually the *Dactylogyridae* and occasionally *Tetraonchidae*. "Coughing" may be the first sign seen, followed by the scraping of their gill covers (operculae) against objects or the sides of the aquarium. As the gills become more severely damaged,

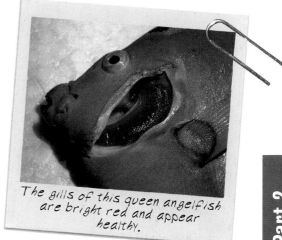

The gills of this queen angelfish are bright red and appear healthy.

heavy, labored breathing will be seen. This includes an increased respiratory rate (faster breathing) with a marked flaring of the operculae.

Irritation caused by the flukes triggers excess mucus production by the gills so that mucus may be seen trailing from the gills. Affected fish may gasp at the surface, especially in areas of high dissolved oxygen such as filter outflows, airstones, and the like. The fish will often refuse to eat and will lose condition as they channel all of their energy into breathing. They may eventually recover or may become so weak and anoxic that they die. These flukes are readily identifiable under the microscope. The most distinguishing features are the hooks at the back end of the fluke that help it attach and four "eye spots" at the "head" end. In most cases the flukes will be moving, but occasionally they may be encapsulated in the gill tissue.

Gill fluke infestations respond well to standard, formalin-containing remedies or to praziquantel as outlined for skin flukes. Reinfestations are common because the egg stage is resistant to chemical attack. This means that repeated treatments at three weekly intervals may be necessary.

Although in theory one could speed up the life cycle by increasing water temperature, thereby exposing the susceptible adults and immature stages to chemical treatment quicker, this would also have the effect of reducing dissolved oxygen levels, which could kill some of your heavily infested fish. If secondary bacterial or fungal infections have established themselves, then these need to be tackled as well.

Any disease damaging the gills or causing a lack of oxygen should be considered, especially if there is a lack of response to specific fluke medication. Poor water quality, such as that including high ammonia, high nitrite, and low oxygen, should be ruled out. Other parasitic gill problems, such as *Chilodonella*, *Trichodina*, *Oodinium*, and *Ichthyophthirius* (white spot), can produce similar signs, as can overdosing with medications such as formalin and malachite green. Bacterial gill disease can mimic a gill fluke infestation, but it can also be a sequel to it.

## Digenetic Trematodes

These are flukes, too, but they have an indirect life cycle, like that of tapeworms. Adults are usually found in the gut of their host but can also be found in other organs such as the liver. The primary host is usually a fish predator such as a bird, reptile, or carnivorous fish.

"Probably the best way to avoid serious problems is to quarantine and prophylactically treat all new stock. Avoiding high stocking levels will reduce the "hit rate" of the free-swimming stages."

Eggs are passed out in the feces and are then eaten by a secondary host—usually an aquatic snail. Here the eggs hatch and develop into the first stage, known as the cercaria stage. The cercariae then abandon their first intermediate host to find a second intermediate host, usually a fish. Sometimes the first intermediate host may be eaten by the second. Typically, cercariae invade the eyes, skin, and muscles of the fish, where they grow into the next stage of metacercariae. The metacercariae can develop into adult trematodes only if eaten by the primary host.

The complex life cycle of digenetic trematodes means that they rarely cause problems in aquaria because there is little or no chance of the life cycle being completed. Where they do occur it is often with wild-caught fish, particularly African and South American fishes and other fishes that are reared outdoors. Livebearers, in particular guppies and swordtails, are frequently parasitized.

### Diagnostic Pointers

A variety of fish species can be parasitized, but it is usually only seen with wild-caught or farm-reared fishes. Multiple small black spots on the skin and deeper in the muscles is characteristic of black spot disease. Blackened cysts appear particularly obvious in light-colored fish such as silver dollars.

*Diplostomulum* selectively targets the lens of the eye and can cause serious eye damage, including cataracts. Designed to make the host fish more vulnerable to predation, this parasite can affect the ability of a fish to see and feed. Unless there are large numbers of cysts, they rarely cause serious problems. Given time, the encysted metacercariae will die off and be replaced by scar tissue.

Treatment is with praziquantel as described for skin flukes. In one study, cestode cysts were eradicated from guppies by the following treatment:
• Treatment in a bath for one hour with a combination of salt, acriflavine, and formalin.
• Treatment in the aquarium with acriflavine and salt only for 36 hours.

# Diseases of Dubious Status

The following diseases may or may not exist as "real" diseases at the time of this writing. It may be that they turn out as syndromes, whereby affected fishes show a range of symptoms and signs. These diseases may be the result of unidentified pathogens such as viruses, or they may be due to a variety of different disease-causing organisms that happen to produce symptoms that may

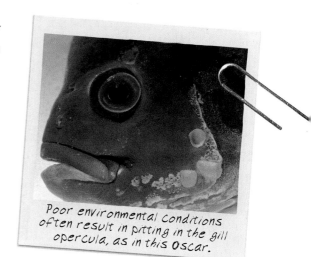

Poor environmental conditions often result in pitting in the gill opercula, as in this Oscar.

overlap with known diseases. I do not make a claim either way but present them because one is likely to come across references to them.

## Malawi Bloat

This is a poorly defined condition that is said to particularly afflict Rift Lake cichlids. It has been attributed to several pathogens, but it is also possible that it is truly caused by a number of different and unrelated conditions. Obvious "bloating" can be due to a buildup of fluid in the abdomen (ascites) as a result of liver, heart, or kidney disease. Often this can be due to bacterial infections, but there are other causes. Toxins released from one bacterium–*Clostridium difficile*–have been linked to Malawi bloat. *Hexamita* can also cause this bloating. In herbivorous fish, any disruption of the normal gut environment (often due to improper diet) can potentially lead to fluid or gas buildup in the intestinal tract. *Cryptobia iubilans* can also cause Malawi bloat if it spreads to the main organs.

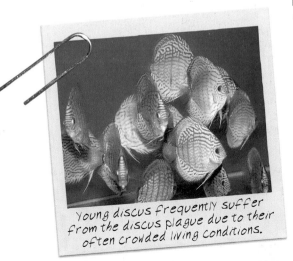

Young discus frequently suffer from the discus plague due to their often crowded living conditions.

## Discus Plague

The typical symptoms of discus plague are lethargy with a darkened coloration and an excessive production of mucus. The breathing rate is often very rapid. Angelfishes *(Pterophyllum* spp.) can also be affected. From a diagnostic point of view, the problem is that these signs may also occur with other known discus diseases such as *Hexamita/Spironucleus* infestations. Sometimes fish can succumb to several diseases at the same time and will show a confusing array of signs

Part 2

that do not appear to fit a "recognized" pattern. If one looks hard enough, *Spironucleus* will often be found, but this does not rule out discus plague.

*Spironucleus*, after all, can be considered a normal inhabitant of the gut of angelfish (and discus), and so you'd probably find it in any case. Infected fish may well show the same signs of disease that are seen with other conditions, but this may be just because fish can only react to many different diseases in a limited number of ways. After being initially skeptical, I have a hunch that there may be something else going on with discus plague– possibly a viral infection. I would argue that more work, including electron microscopy, needs to be done on suspected cases before a conclusion can be reached.

## Black Spot Disease Of Hybrid Parrot Cichlids

Hybrid parrot cichlids are said to occasionally succumb to "black spot" disease. The color patterns can be variable in these fish, and so black markings can come and go over time. Deaths suffered while fish are showing these "black spots" may be due to other diseases such as *Spironucleus*, with the altered coloration being incidental. Having said that, *Oreochromis mossambicus* infected with one type of fish-TB (*Mycobacterium marinum*) did develop areas of melanin concentration around inflamed areas of the skin (and in some internal organs) as part of their response to this infection. This produced small, black-pigmented areas in the skin. However, this effect appears to be an uncommon one. Another possibility is that it could be *Plistophora* triggering melanocyte accumulations, as it appears to do in angelfish. Again, more work needs to be done on this condition if it is to be resolved.

## Dropsy (Ascites and Oedema)

Dropsy is not a disease in its own right but a serious symptom or sign that can come about from a variety of different diseases and disorders.

Unfortunately, in many hobbyist texts and on proprietary treatment instructions, it is often erroneously considered to be a distinct disease in its own right.

Dropsy is more correctly termed **ascites**, a condition in which there is a buildup of fluid inside the body cavities of the fish. **Oedema** occurs when fluid actually collects within the fish's tissues. When this fluid accumulates in the main body cavity (known as the coelom), what we see is a swelling or ballooning out of the body wall. This fluid, which is under some pressure due to the limitations of the space within the coelom, compresses the internal organs and blood vessels. This is how it affects the normal functioning of these organs. Fluid also infiltrates into the microscopic spaces in the tissues around the scales, causing an obvious protrusion of the scales to give the characteristic "pinecone" appearance associated with dropsy.

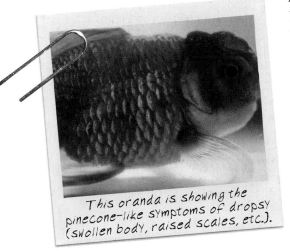

*This oranda is showing the pinecone-like symptoms of dropsy (swollen body, raised scales, etc.).*

These fluid accumulations form because the fish is unable to control its fluid and salt balance with the surrounding water. To better explain why this fluid accumulation takes place, we need to take a step back and look at some of the problems encountered by fishes living in fresh water.

The fluids inside a fish (such as blood and lymph) are relatively more concentrated than the surrounding water because they have a wide variety of substances dissolved in them. Examples of these would be blood proteins, hormones, and salts. Fish skin and gill tissue are freely permeable to tiny water molecules, which can slip through the microscopic gaps between cells. Larger molecules such as proteins cannot do this. Because the skin acts as a barrier to only some molecules, it may be regarded as a partially permeable barrier.

Water molecules are constantly moving across this partially permeable barrier into the fish in an effort to dilute its more concentrated internal fluids. This is known as **osmosis**, and the partially permeable barrier can be referred to as an osmotic barrier. It is vitally important that many of the substances found in the blood and other body fluids have their concentrations controlled within very tight limits. The fish must therefore actively take account of the constant diluting effect of osmosis by excreting excess water (or salts if the concentration is too high) out of its system to keep the status quo. This regulation is called, not surprisingly, **osmoregulation.**

The main organs involved with osmoregulation are the gills, the kidneys (freshwater fish produce large volumes of dilute urine), and to a lesser extent, the intestines. If those organs used in osmoregulation are damaged or otherwise unable to function, then there can be a buildup of fluid inside the fish. The cause of dropsy is usually a multifactorial condition, with disease processes going on in several different organs at once.

Any disease process that interferes with osmoregulation in freshwater fish can result in an overall accumulation of fluid in the fish that will, in turn, manifest itself as the signs of dropsy. Common examples of these are:
• Heart disease
• Liver disease
• Gill diseases such as ectoparasites (like *Dactylogyrus*)
• Bacterial gill disease and fungal infections
• Kidney diseases, including mycobacterial infections (fish tuberculosis)

Part 2

- Protozoal parasites like *Hoferellus carassii* in goldfish
- Noninfectious disorders, such as polycystic disease, again in goldfish
- Gut disorders, including severe parasitism by worms or protozoa (for example, coccidia)

## Heart Disease

Heart disease is the failure of the heart to effectively pump blood around the circulatory system, which can seriously affect how well various organs function. In addition, pooling of blood in veins because it is not being circulated properly can lead to fluid leaking out of these blood vessels into surrounding spaces and so contribute to the problem.

Ulceration or any breach in the partially permeable barrier can allow a major inrush of water to swamp the fishes' normal osmoregulatory balance. This can have other serious consequences by allowing the loss of proteins and salts from the body, as they can bypass the osmotic barrier.

## Liver Disease

One of the many jobs of the liver is to manufacture proteins that are required in the blood stream. These proteins are large molecules; because their presence bumps up the overall concentration of the blood, they have an effect on osmosis. If the liver is not functioning properly, then these proteins may not be produced in sufficient quantity. This means that there is less difference between the concentration of the blood inside the blood vessel and the fluid in the surrounding tissues than there should be. This results in water molecules leaving the blood and accumulating in the surrounding tissues and spaces.

## What to Look For

Any freshwater species is likely to be affected. Most often, a swollen body cavity accompanied by classic "pine cone" outline will lead one to this

**Part 2**

Part 2

diagnosis. Other signs such as ulceration, hemorrhage, loss of balance due to compression of the swim bladder, and heavy breathing may be seen.

Remember that "dropsy" is only a sign of disease, and consideration must be given as to what the underlying problem is. Do not stop at dropsy as a diagnosis–investigate further to try to find out why it is occurring. *Dropsy is not a diagnosis in its own right!*

## Treatment

Attempt to identify underlying problems and treat for them. Because the accumulation of fluid within the fish is due to osmosis, reducing the difference in concentration between the fluids inside the fish and the water around it may help to redress the balance. This can be done by adding pure salt or sea salt to increase the water's concentration. A 0.3% salt solution is ideal–this equates to 30g (around 2 tablespoons) of salt added to every 10 liters of aquarium water, or 3.0kg per 1,000 liters of pond water. Drawing off fluid from the coelom by syringe and needle is sometimes of benefit. However, there are dangers in attempting this, including:

• The risk of damaging the internal organs with the needle if one is unfamiliar with the internal anatomy of that fish species

• One may be removing vital dissolved substances along with the fluid so that the fish may die of shock following such an invasive procedure.

• The risk of introducing infection into the body cavity of the fish.

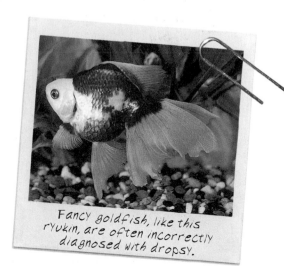

Fancy goldfish, like this ryukin, are often incorrectly diagnosed with dropsy.

• Sedation (it is best to perform this procedure under sedation), for example with oil of cloves, is an extra stress on an already compromised fish, and so there is an increased risk of the fish dying.

By the time a fish is showing obvious signs of dropsy, it is a very sick individual indeed, with the odds of recovery heavily stacked against it. It may also be acting as a reservoir of infection for your other fish. If you cannot hospitalize it in a separate aquarium or vat for treatment, I would strongly urge you to consider euthanasia of the fish on humane grounds. Dropsy may seem like a condition that can be readily identified, but there are some conditions for which it can be mistaken. Internal tumors are the most likely problem to cause confusion, but the body outline of such fish is often not symmetrical, and usually the scales do not protrude. Other internal abnormalities such as polycystic kidneys in goldfish can cause swelling of the body cavity, but again without scale protrusion.

SVC is sometimes called infectious dropsy because of the characteristic swelling of the abdomen. Other signs include hemorrhages in the skin and mucoid faecal casts or strings hanging from an often protruding vent. At first glance one could be forgiven for confusing pearl-scale goldfish, with their globular bodies and raised scales, with a severe case of dropsy!

# Medicines, Sedation, and Euthanasia

It is an obvious statement, but diagnosis of a disease is only part of the way to solving your problem. To completely solve the problem, you will often need to medicate with an appropriate treatment. For successful medication, you need to have as accurate a diagnosis as possible. Keep in mind that all medications work selectively— there is no "cure-all." This means that treating with a medication

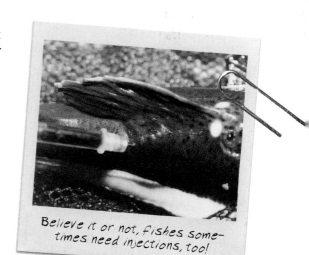

Believe it or not, fishes sometimes need injections, too!

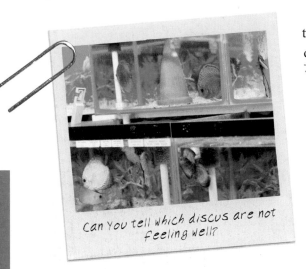

Can you tell which discus are not feeling well?

that is not designed for the specific disease that your fishes have will not work. This is probably the main cause of treatment failures. A common scenario is for hobbyists to gradually work their way along the whole shelf of preparations available in their local aquarium shop, one or two at a time, without making any real attempt to arrive at a diagnosis. At best, incorrect treatments are useless–just a waste of time and money. At worst, they can turn a difficult situation into a crisis. Without laboratory diagnostics, most of us work on a "best guess" basis, but by using the information and the Diagnostic Pointers provided in the previous sections, you can go a long way toward achieving an accurate diagnosis.

Always treat a disease with the correct concentration or amount of medication. This particularly applies to antibiotics. Using dosages that are too low will help to select for resistant strains of bacteria, resulting in antibiotics once very useful such as oxytetracycline becoming useless in many cases. Also, it's important to treat for an appropriate length of time. Many parasites have life cycles lasting several weeks, and so treatment may be needed for at least that amount of time, if not more. Some, such as gill flukes, have resistant egg or cyst stages, meaning that repeated treatments are necessary. In addition, medicate in an appropriate form. For example, simply adding medication to the water can easily treat external parasites, but internal problems may need medication to be given in food, by injection, and/or by stomach tube. Finally, some fish are naturally sensitive to certain medications, so always try to find alternatives. Just lowering the dose rate may seem sensible, but you are probably only helping the pathogen by doing so!

## Treatment Methods
### In the Aquarium or Pond

This is the easiest option for the common fishkeeper. It has some advantages for the fish as well, such as less stress, and the water quality is likely to remain optimal. Unfortunately, some medications are not in an appropriate water-soluble form or are too expensive to use in large volumes. Worse still, some medications, like antibiotics, can affect biological filters by destroying the filter bacteria, or they can affect other inhabitants of the same body of water. Formalin, for example, will effectively kill off swan mussels introduced into ponds. Always remove carbon filtration if medication is added to the water.

### In a Treatment or Quarantine Area

The advantages of this are that treatment is in smaller, known volumes. The main pond or aquarium is protected from any harmful effects of the medication. The fish may find it more stressful, but this does not outweigh the advantages.

### As a Bath

Fish are placed in a small volume of water for a relatively short period of time. This involves catching the fish on a regular basis and potentially repeatedly stressing it, but again it means that no medication needs to be put into the main pond or aquarium.

### In Food

This theory is very simple, but problems arise because sick fish often do not eat or do not eat enough, or they may be out-competed by healthier fish and so not get any medication. Many drugs and chemicals are not suitable to be incorporated into food.

### By Injection

Please seek assistance and ask to be shown how to do this first before attempting it. The advantage of the injection is that the amount of drug delivered is accurate; the disadvantage is that fish must be caught up first, and some fish may be too small to inject.

### By Stomach Tube

This is a good way of giving some drugs to large fish. Use a soft tube (ask your veterinarian or a pharmacist for advice on which type) and gently pass it down the gullet of the fish. As with injections, an accurate amount is given, but again the fish must be caught and possibly sedated to allow you to do this. If the tube misses the gullet, it may damage the gills.

## Proprietary Medicines

A great number of proprietary, off-the-shelf medications are available for ornamental fishes. The simple fact is that many just do not work as effectively as the blurb on the packaging leads us to expect. This is due to a number of factors, one of which is that the manufacturers are only able to use products that are not tightly controlled by legislation because they are deemed to be "safe." This categorization varies from country to country, but as an example, few if any antibiotics are legally available over-the-counter. As a rough guide, treatments for white spot and other external parasites often work very well, while those deemed appropriate for bacterial infections often perform poorly. Most of the preparations available today are mixtures and variations on those mixtures of the following chemicals.

### Malachite Green

This medication is a very effective antifungal and antiectoparasiticide. In the United Kingdom, its use on fishes reared for human consumption has been banned. It is, however, still legal to use it for ornamental fish providing you do not eat them afterward. Overdose affects fish at a cellular level and causes symptoms in the fish like that of oxygen starvation, even if there is plenty of oxygen available. Malachite green is more toxic at temperatures above 21$^O$C. Tetras and scaleless fish such as morymids and botias are particularly suseptible.

**Dose rates for Malachite Green:**
• 0.1mg/liter as a permanent bath
• 2mg/liter for 30 minutes. Repeat daily for 3 days.
• 50-60mg/liter baths for 10 to 30 seconds. Repeat this three times every day for three days.

## Methylene Blue

A useful medication for its effects against the free-swimming larval stages of white spot, it may help the release of stored red blood cells from the spleen. It can harm biological filters.

**Dose:** 2mg/liter as a prolonged bath, up to 48 hours.

## Acriflavine

**Dose rates:**
5 to 10mg/liter as a prolonged bath, repeated once daily to effect.
500mg/liter as a half hour bath repeated once daily to effect.

## Salt

Often acts as a mild pick-me-up, although some fish such as *Corydoras* spp. are said to be sensitive to it.

**Dose rates:**
1-5g/liter as a permanent bath
30-35g/liter as a five-minute bath

## Formalin

May also be quoted as formaldehyde. The dose rates given are based on the use of full- strength formalin that is 37% formaldehyde. Do not use if

**Part 2**

there are white bits in it, as these will be precipitates of toxic paraformaldehyde. Make sure the water is well aerated when using formalin. It is more toxic in soft and acidic water and at higher temperatures, so opt for lower doses.

**Dose rates:**

0.125-0.25ml/liter as a bath for up to 60 minutes, repeated every 24 hours for two to three days.

0.015-0.025ml/liter as a permanent bath. Repeat every two days for a total of six days.

## Quinine Hydrochloride

This is safe with scaleless fish such as *Botia* and mormyrids.

**Dose rate:** 1.5g/liter for two to three days

## Povidone-iodine

This is applied directly to open wounds as an antibacterial and antifungal cleanser.

## Copper-based Medications

These are a good ectoparasiticide, but can is toxic to invertebrates and stingrays. They are used particularly with marine aquarium fish. Monitor copper levels using commercially available test kits, maintaining the free copper levels at 0.15 to 0.2mg/liter until therapeutic effect is obtained.

## Benzalkonium Chloride

This is a surfactant. The toxicity of benzalkonium chloride is increased in soft water, and doses should be reduced if the water is soft or if softness not known.

**Dose rates:**

10mg/liter as a five to ten minute bath

5mg/liter for a 30-minute bath

Part 2

2mg/liter for a 60-minute bath

1mg/liter for several hours

## Potassium Permanganate

Bath at 10ppm (mg/l) for 5 to 60 minutes can be used to rid both individual fish and plants of parasites. Do not use with formalin.

## Leteux-Meyer Formulation

This is a combination of malachite green at 3.3g/liter and formalin at 0.015ml/liter. This is changed every 48 hours for a total of three treatments.

## Combinations

Salt, formalin, and acriflavine have been used in combination to eradicate cestode cysts from guppies, as well as skin and gill flukes, white spot, *Trichodina*, and *Oodinium*. A suggested regime would be:

Treatment in a bath for one hour with a combination of salt (10g/liter), acriflavine (10mg/liter), and formalin (0.2mls/liter).

Treatment in the aquarium with acriflavine (5mg/liter) and salt (5mg/liter) only for 36 hours.

# Veterinary Medications

The next groups of drugs are those that in the majority of countries are controlled to some extent. Often they are only available through a veterinarian or pharmacist. These controls are there primarily to prevent incorrect use of them or because they may be hazardous to use.

All fish undergoing treatment should be kept at their optimum temperature. Not only will this encourage recovery, but it also ensures normal metabolic handling of medications, such as elimination from the body by the kidneys or liver.

Part 2

## Antibiotics

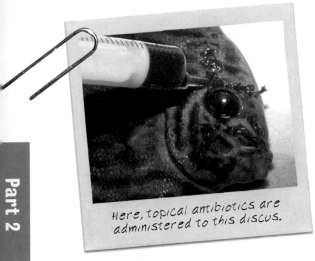

Here, topical antibiotics are administered to this discus.

Antibiotics are often used in ornamental fish, but few, if any, are licensed for use in these species. The common problems with antibiotics are that they are often present in a form unsuitable for easy administration to fish (e.g. as injectables or tablets) that must be modified to try to make them suitable for medicating fish. Mixing antibiotic powder with food can be done, but sick fish often do not feed. Injection is another option, but it is a skill that needs to be taught by an experienced fish health professional, and some owners may just not be able to handle doing it.

In the majority of countries, the supply of antibiotics is tightly controlled, and this can make it difficult and expensive to access them. Those antibiotics that are freely available, such as oxytetracycline in some countries, often fail to perform because there is widespread bacterial resistance to them as a direct result of their uncontrolled usage.

Adding an antibiotic directly to an aquarium or pond is likely to damage the biological filtration and so create serious water-quality problems.

Antibiotic safety and efficacy has only been investigated for a small number of commercially important species, such as trout and salmon, so their use on the wide range of ornamental species may carry some risks.

### Enrofloxacin
**Injection:** 5-10mg/kg every 48 hours for 15 days
**Bath:** 2.5mg/l as a five-hour bath every 24 hours for five to seven days
**Infeed:** 5mg/kg of fish daily for 10-14 days.

### Potentiated Sulphonamides
**Injection:** 30mg/kg every 24 hours for seven to ten days
**Infeed:** 30mg/kg of fish every 24 hrs for 10-14 days

### Oxolinic Acid
**Infeed:** 10mg/kg of fish daily for ten days

### Oxytetracycline
Oxytetracycline is chelated by hard water. This inactivates the antibiotic, so higher doses need to be used in hard water. Oxytetracycline has been used so extensively over the years that there is much bacterial resistance to it. At higher dose rates (e.g. 40mg/kg by injection), it may be immunosuppressive.
**Injection:** 10mg/kg daily for 10-14 days
**Bath:** 100mg/l for one hour daily for five to ten days
**Infeed:** 75mg/kg daily for 7-14 days

### Metronidazole
This can be used to treat protozoan infestations as well as metronidazole-sensitive bacterial infections.
**Bath:** <50mg/l daily for up to 24 hours for ten days
**Infeed:** 100mg/kg of fish daily for ten days

### Chloramphenicol
Rarely used these days, in fish it may be immunosuppressive if used over long periods.
Inject at 40mg/kg once daily.

## Wormers
### Praziquantel
For discus and smaller tropicals, a suggested dosage method with praziquantel is a one to two hour bath at 15-20mg/l.

With larger fish such as koi, infeeding medication at a rate of 400mg/100g food daily for seven days would be more appropriate.

### Levamisole
This is particularly good for killing larval worms. Suspend carbon filtration. 10mg/l as a single dose added to the water.

### Piperazine
2.5mg/g of feed, added to the food. This may only kill adult worms.

### Fenbendazole
50mg/kg bodyweight added to feed or by stomach tube if the fish is large enough.

### Lufrenon
Lufrenon is most often used as a flea-control agent in dogs and cats. It works by affecting the ability of immature stages of crustaceans like *Argulus* to molt correctly, thereby causing their death. It is not licensed for use on fish. It must only be used for ornamental fish. The product is thought to be quite persistent in the environment, and I would not recommend its use in natural ponds, where serious damage to the pond's ecology could occur. It is best used at a dose of 0.088mg/liter as a once only treatment.

### Organophosphates
Organophosphates have in the past been a significant weapon in our arsenal against fish parasites, especially flukes and crustaceans. Due to

environmental concerns, they have become very tightly controlled in countries such the UK. Resistance to organophosphates has been recorded in some populations of flukes.

One organophosphate that is available in many countries is trichlorophon. Suggested dose rates are:
• 0.5mg/liter as a permanent bath. Give three treatments over a period of ten days.
• 0.5mg/liter as a permanent bath. Give four treatments over seven days for anchor worm and flukes.

## Sedation

Popular among hobbyists and available as a commercial product, clove oil is usually used as a sedative for larger fish. There appears to be no particular dose rate for clove oil, and there is a varied susceptibility among individual fish.

Add 1ml of clove oil into 2 gallons of water in a bag. This should be shaken vigorously and left for five to ten minutes with the bag sealed as tightly as possible. This provides your anesthetic solution. Add incrementally to effect. Recovery will occur when the fish is returned to clean water.

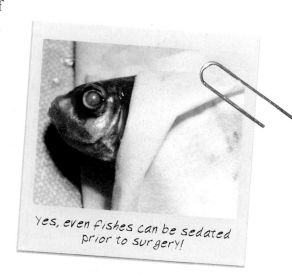

Yes, even fishes can be sedated prior to surgery!

## Euthanasia

With some sick fish, euthanasia may be the only humane act that you can perform for it. The best ways for the hobbyist to undertake this are still

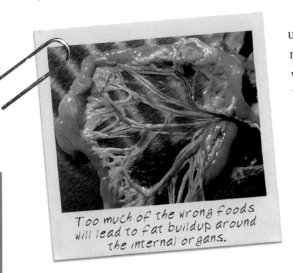

Too much of the wrong foods will lead to fat buildup around the internal organs.

uncertain, and you will get different responses from different people. One way is to overdose with clove oil. This will put the fish to sleep in a very effective and humane manner. Another method often used is to place the fish in a small volume of water and add as many as possible. As these tablets fizz, carbon dioxide is released, which in turn forms carbonic acid. This results in an overdose of carbon dioxide, and the fish will pass peacefully. Be aware that an unsightly scum is often left on the surface of the water.

Methods of euthanasia to avoid include the decapitation of a fish without prior stunning. Be aware that fish nerve tissue is tolerant of anoxia, and the brain may continue to function for some time after decapitation. Freezing is a method favored by many hobbyists, but many fish are able to cope with very low temperatures. Remember that just because a fish cannot respond to a stimulus when hypothermic does not guarantee that it cannot perceive it. Either way, it is probably best to ask your local veterinarian for his or her recommendations, and always consult local fish/wildlife services, as some forms of euthanasia are considered to be cruel and are outlawed in many areas.

## Quarantine

Quarantining of new fish is an important barrier against the introduction of infectious disease into an established collection. Unfortunately, it is a fact that few hobbyists do practice quarantine procedures. This is a shame, because despite what you may believe, few retailers or wholesalers quarantine their fish before they go on sale. This is largely a commercial decision because they may not have the space needed to quarantine large numbers of fish. In addition, there may be some reluctance to pass on to the consumer the extra costs that quarantining entails–feeding fish and keeping them warm costs money.

I would strongly argue that the advantages of quarantining far outweigh any argument against a quarantining period, so let's take a look at what is involved in quarantining at home. In its simplest form, it involves keeping new fish in complete isolation from the main collection for a period of time. Freshwater tropical and coldwater fish are kept in normal glass or acrylic aquaria, while vats are commonly used for the larger pond fish.

One of the most common hitches with quarantining is failing to provide optimal water quality. A small acrylic container clipped to the inside of the aquarium is just not adequate. If you do not look after your quarantine facility properly, then any quarantined fish are likely to sicken while in quarantine–an ironic situation. To get the full benefit from quarantining, I would suggest that you keep all heaters, nets, and other equipment used with your quarantine setup completely separate from those used with your other aquaria or ponds.

Quarantine facilities should be as basic as possible to allow accurate

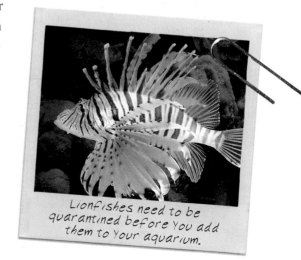

Lionfishes need to be quarantined before you add them to your aquarium.

Part 2

volume estimation for dosing with medication. Water-quality parameters (including temperature) should be optimal for the species. Filtration should be provided, but you cannot rely upon biological filtration, as medications may destroy these bacteria. Also, after every quarantine period, the aquarium or vat should be dismantled and sterilized with an iodine-based disinfectant. No trace of iodine must be left before setting up again. You therefore cannot use biological filtration, which takes time to establish. Some aquarists keep a few small fish in the quarantine system to keep the biological filter functioning, but then there is a risk that these fish may be disease carriers, helping to infect your quarantine facility.

## Pros of Quarantining New Fishes

• New fish have often received individual attention. Therefore, these fish are fitter and better able to compete when introduced to their final home.

• It allows new fish time to adjust to new water conditions and management regimes such as differing foods, different day/night cycles, and so on.

• Any disease that the fish may be carrying is liable to manifest itself during the quarantine period, giving you a chance to treat it before your main collection is put at risk.

• Any medications used are in a situation safely removed from your main collection and biological filtration.

## Cons of Quarantining New Fishes

• Extra space is required for the quarantine aquaria or vats.

• Quarantine facilities should be large enough to comfortably house the largest fish that you are likely to buy.

• For quarantine facilities to work properly, water quality in the quarantine facility should be as good as in your main display.

• You lose the instant gratification of seeing the fish that you have just bought swimming in your main display.

Without biological filtration, you need to rely upon physical and chemical methods of water purification. Zeolite can be used to absorb ammonia excreted by the fish, and the use of activated charcoal will adsorb many harmful chemicals from the water. Ozonizers and ultraviolet sterilization would also be appropriate. Keep decorations to a minimum, simply providing a sufficient

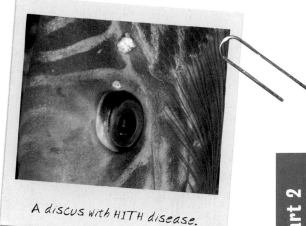

A discus with HITH disease.

amount for nervous fish to hide behind. All materials used for quarantine should be readily cleanable (for example, plastic). Avoid live plants and bogwood, which can possibly act as disease reservoirs.

The length of time for which you should quarantine your fish will vary according to which diseases concern you. I would suggest a minimum of 2 weeks (preferably 4) for all fish, with this extending to 8 to 12 weeks for coldwater fish when kept at lower temperature ranges (because most diseases will take longer to manifest at these temperatures).

In general, I would not suggest routine medications, as many treatments can be stressful to the fish. The exception to this would be to treat all freshwater fish for white spot, as it is so ubiquitous.

# Index

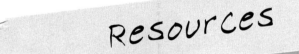

## Publications

**Tropical Fish Hobbyist Magazine**
1 TFH Plaza
Third & Union Avenues
Neptune City, NJ 07753
Telephone: (800) 631-2188
E-mail: Info@tfhpublications.com
www.tfhpublications.com

## Organizations

**Federation of American Aquarium Societies (FAAS)**
Secretary: Jane Benes
E-mail: Jbenes01@yahoo.com
www.gcca.net/faas

**Federation of British Aquatic Societies (FBAS)**
Secretary: Vivienne Pearce
E-mail: Webmaster@fbas.co.uk
www.fbas.co.uk

## Internet Resources

**AquaLink**
(www.aqualink.com)
The largest aquaria web resource in the world, AquaLink provides fishkeepers with information on a variety of topics, including freshwater and marine fish, aquatic plants, goldfish, reef systems, invertebrates, and corals.